Healing
Signs

Healing Signs

The Astrological Guide to Wholeness and Well-Being

RONNIE GALE DREYER

MAIN
STREET
BOOKS

DOUBLEDAY
New York   London   Toronto
Sydney   Auckland

A MAIN STREET BOOK

PUBLISHED BY DOUBLEDAY

a division of Random House, Inc.

1540 Broadway, New York, New York 10036

MAIN STREET BOOKS, DOUBLEDAY, and the portrayal of a building with a
tree are trademarks of Doubleday, a division of Random House, Inc.

BOOK DESIGN BY DEBORAH KERNER

Reflexology Chart copyright © 1991 by Gordon Russell. Used by permission of Two Steps
to Health. Acupressure points reproduced by permission of Gaia Books Ltd., from *Acupressure for Common Ailments* by Chris Jarmey and John Tindall, illustrated by Allison
Champion. Call 00 44 (0) 1453 752985 for further information. Illustrations of yoga poses
by Judith DuFour Love.

Library of Congress Cataloging-in-Publication Data

Dreyer, Ronnie Gale.
Healing signs: the astrological guide to wholeness and well-being /
by Ronnie Gale Dreyer. — 1st ed.
p. cm.
Includes bibliographical references and index.
1. Astrology and health. I. Title.
BF1729.H9D74 2000
133.2′8613—dc21 99-40920
CIP

ISBN 0-385-49815-2
Copyright © 2000 by Ronnie Gale Dreyer
All Rights Reserved
Printed in the United States of America
February 2000
First Edition
10 9 8 7 6 5 4 3 2 1

Acknowledgments

I would like to thank the following people for their invaluable contributions to *Healing Signs:* my agent, Bob Silverstein, for his persistence and encouragement; my editor at Doubleday, Jennifer Griffin, for her attention to detail, a gentle yet firm helping hand, and, thankfully, the ability to push me to the absolute limits; Madalyn Hillis-Dineen and Ray White of Astrolabe, Inc., for taking time out of their busy schedules to supply and format the charts and ephemerides used in this book; Randi Jurgens, R.N.C., for answering many of my medical questions; my husband, Ken Irving, for editorial advice, love, support, and belief in me; and Fran Dreyer for editing, proofreading, and assisting me, often at very short notice, with whatever needed to be done, from research to hand holding. Without her help, this book would never have reached completion. As always, I'd like to thank my friends, family, students, and clients from whom I continue to learn each day and, finally, the healers, medical practitioners, therapists, astrologers, and teachers with whom I have worked and consulted over the years, and who are too numerous to mention. I do owe a special debt of gratitude to the late Ira Progoff, whose *Intensive Journal* method provided me and thousands of others a new way of dialoging with the inner self. If I have learned anything at all from my mentors, it is to continue questioning, to enjoy life to the fullest, and, above all, to know and heal thyself whenever possible.

Contents

ix

Contents

Introduction

Holistic healing, or treating the entire individual rather than just the symptoms, has entered mainstream America. Treatments once considered alternative, even quackery, are being embraced by the general population and are slowly infiltrating the medical establishment. More and more doctors, nurses, and therapists are concurring that nontraditional healing techniques are beneficial and are recommending them in conjunction with orthodox medicine. Acupuncture, yoga, massage therapy, and chiropractic services are just some of the claims now reimbursed by many insurance companies, and books whose subjects range from the powers of the mind to aromatherapy to spiritual healing consistently top the best-seller lists. To further validate the growing interest in holistic medicine, the National Center for Complementary and Alternative Medicine (NCCAM) has been established as part of the National Institutes of Health to provide the public with information on alternative healing methods. More and more people are exploring the large variety of healing options that natural and alternative medicine offer.

While some may think that these healing methods are revolutionary, in fact, most ancient cultures utilized natural healing methods as a way of curing illness and relieving pain in the quest to achieve healthy living. The Chinese have practiced acupuncture for over five thousand years. Native Americans and Egyptians have always relied on potent indigenous herbs to cure mental and physical illness. Yoga, massage, and Ayurvedic medicine have been essential to healing in India for centuries and are listed extensively in the Vedas, the Hindu equivalent of the Bible. Europeans have always been strong believers in homeopathic medicine in response to a common belief that illness is psychosomatic, that is, the state of the mind is linked to the condition of the body.

According to holistic practitioners, the key to maintaining good health lies in strengthening the immune system, the body's defense mechanism, by preventing mental, emotional, and physical stress from wearing it down so that viruses, bacteria, or other intruders cannot attack. Haven't you ever noticed that no matter how much vitamin C you ingest during the winter cold season, you will nonetheless become ill if you are overworked and your energy depleted? After all, emotional anxiety, fatigue, and depression wear down the ability to fight illness—the body's way of saying that the immune system is weak and requires rest in order for it to be energized. Holistic medicine can restore health and prevent disease. Massage, for example, a stress management technique which is inexpensive and relatively safe, may prevent the onset of backache by relaxing and stretching the muscles. If discomfort or pain has already set in, massage may soothe aching joints and muscles by increasing blood flow and oxygen to the afflicted areas.

When your emotional and physical stamina are in optimum condition, your body produces endorphins, chemicals that create a feeling of well-being. You can achieve this elevated state by us-ing a plethora of techniques yourself or with the help of a pro-fessional. The holistic practitioner will give you a thorough physical examination, then inquire about your moods, habits, likes and dislikes to ascertain if an ailment is directly linked to your state of mind. Questions to determine your preferences as to cold or warm climates, spicy or bland foods, etc., are not un-common to categorize your personality type.

Learning to relax mind and body in a stress-free environment will help you avoid ailments such as indigestion, headache, fa-tigue, muscle strain, and backache, to name a few. Chronic con-ditions including asthma, arthritis, cancer, and colitis may also be treated with both traditional medicine and holistic tech-niques. Acupuncture, for example, is now recognized by the Na-tional Institutes of Health as a method for relieving arthritic pain. While it is not a complete panacea, acupuncture has been effective in making life bearable and even productive for arthri-tis sufferers by reducing pain and restoring mobility.

Heart disease is a prime example of an illness to which you may be naturally predisposed but can ward off before it becomes life-threatening. You can take control of your heart's health by al-tering your lifestyle to include a low-fat diet, aerobic exercise, and stress reduction, that is, using the power of the mind to con-trol the reactions of your body. If you already have a heart con-dition, health consciousness and lifestyle changes are not only recommended but required by cardiologists, along with ortho-dox medication.

Throughout this book we will be utilizing astrology, the interre-lationship between celestial activity and mundane events, to im-prove our ability to prevent illness before it occurs. Since our signs are the key to our physical and psychological makeups, the more we know about our strengths and vulnerabilities through astrology, the easier it may be to treat illness.

The following chapters are classified according to sign in order for you to judge the best way each sign may prevent and combat illnesses to which you may be prone.

Chapter 1

How the Stars
Affect Your Health

———————◆———————

The Magical Moment of Birth:
Your Personal Horoscope
as Your Genetic Marker

If you took a snapshot of the sky at the moment you inhaled
your very first breath, you would have a photograph of the
Sun, Moon, and the eight planets* against a backdrop of the
twelve constellations into which our galaxy is divided (as seen
from the Earth). Known as the zodiacal belt or, more commonly,
the twelve signs of the zodiac, these groupings were first cited
and named by the ancient Babylonians, who viewed the heavens
as a series of pictures the stars seemed to form. The first cluster
of stars reminded them of a ram, which they named Aries, followed by other picturesque groups that they sequentially called
Taurus the Bull, Gemini the Twins, Cancer the Crab, Leo the
Lion, Virgo the Virgin, Libra the Scales, Scorpio the Scorpion,

---

*Because we view the movements of the luminaries from the perspective of being on Earth, the
eight planets are Mercury, Venus, Mars, Jupiter, Saturn, Uranus, Neptune, and Pluto. For astrological purposes, the Sun and Moon, known to the ancients as the "lights," are also regarded as
planets.

5

Sagittarius the Archer, Capricorn the Goat, Aquarius the Water Bearer, and Pisces the Fish (Fig. 1.1).

The Sun, Moon, and planets, which travel through the zodiacal belt, were worshiped by the ancients as celestial deities. Surrounded by the magnificent constellations, the ancient skies must have resembled a great stage where, night after night, the skirmishes and romances of their gods and goddesses were dramatized before their very eyes.

If you are fortunate enough to observe the sky on a clear evening with the aid of a telescope, or even with the naked eye, you can see the constellational shapes and sizes as distinctly as did the ancient Babylonians, Egyptians, Indians, Persians, and Greeks. Since the Sun is visible only during daylight hours, and the stars come out only at night, it is impossible to see the Sun against the backdrop of its constellation unless the sky is viewed at sunrise or sunset, when the Sun and the stars are equally visible. However, you will be able to see the Moon and some of the planets in their zodiacal signs most evenings. Of course, the time of year and your location will determine which planets can be viewed with the naked eye and which ones will need to be seen with the aid of a telescope.

Each planet's position in its zodiacal sign and its relationship to the other planets at the moment of birth form the basis of the horoscope. Derived from the Greek *hora,* meaning "hour," and *scope,* meaning "picture" or "vision," the horoscope is an image of the heavens at the exact time and place of birth and what astrologers believe spells out the story of your life.

Just as heredity defines much of who you are prior to conditioning by home, school, and society, astrology may be said to serve the same purpose. Since each planet represents a different aspect of human nature, the planets may be viewed as genetic

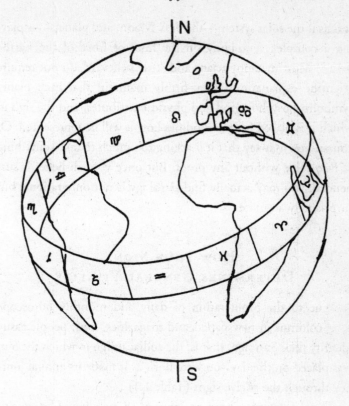

FIGURE I.I I2 SIGNS OF THE ZODIAC

markers which, based on their position and relationship to one another, predispose you to certain character traits, physical conditions, and, ultimately, illnesses.

This concept is supported by some scientists and astronomers, who theorize that at the moment of birth we are affected by the magnetic fields of the Earth and the Sun, which "are bound up with the positions and movements of the planets.

It is as if the solar system—the Sun, Moon, and planets—is playing a complex symphony on the lines of force of the Earth's field."[1] Most metaphysicians and "true believers" do not require scientific explanations; they firmly maintain that each planet symbolizes psychological and physical attributes, and the sign in which it is placed further modifies how it will be represented. Of course, you may say that it is asking too much to take something at face value without any proof. But once your disbelief is suspended, you may actually find astrology is not only rational but surprisingly accurate.

How Your Sign
Determines General Vitality

Due to the proliferation of daily and monthly horoscope columns in newspapers and magazines, most people easily identify their Sun sign, that is, the zodiacal sign in which the Sun was placed on the day you were born as it made its annual journey through the twelve signs (Table 1.1).

Thus, if you were born on January 28, you would be considered an Aquarius since the Sun passes through the sign of Aquarius between January 20 and February 18. Going one step further, it is easy to see on which degree your Sun falls by simply advancing the date one degree per day. Since January 20 represents zero degrees of Aquarius, your Sun would be situated at 8 degrees Aquarius if you were born on January 28.

While the Moon, Mercury, and the remainder of the planets also fell in one of the signs on the day you were born, they may or may not have been positioned in the same sign as your Sun. Like the Sun, the planets are constantly on the move, albeit at different rates of speed and, therefore, their precise positions change daily. Whereas the Sun takes an entire year to travel

Table 1.1 ◆ Twelve Signs of the Zodiac

ZODIACAL SIGN	GLYPH	DATE	RULING PLANET & GLYPH		ELEMENT	MODALITY
Aries	♈	*March 21–April 19*	*Mars*	♂	*Fire*	*Cardinal*
Taurus	♉	*April 20–May 20*	*Venus*	♀	*Earth*	*Fixed*
Gemini	♊	*May 21–June 22*	*Mercury*	☿	*Air*	*Mutable*
Cancer	♋	*June 23–July 22*	*Moon*	☽	*Water*	*Cardinal*
Leo	♌	*July 23–August 22*	*Sun*	☉	*Fire*	*Fixed*
Virgo	♍	*August 23–September 20*	*Mercury*	☿	*Earth*	*Mutable*
Libra	♎	*September 21–October 22*	*Venus*	♀	*Air*	*Cardinal*
Scorpio	♏	*October 23–November 22*	*Pluto* *Mars*	♇ ♂ *(coruler)*	*Water*	*Fixed*
Sagittarius	♐	*November 23–December 20*	*Jupiter*	♃	*Fire*	*Mutable*
Capricorn	♑	*December 21–January 19*	*Saturn*	♄	*Earth*	*Cardinal*
Aquarius	♒	*January 20–February 18*	*Uranus* *Saturn*	♅ ♄ *(coruler)*	*Air*	*Fixed*
Pisces	♓	*February 19–March 20*	*Neptune* *Jupiter*	♆ ♃ *(coruler)*	*Water*	*Mutable*

through the twelve signs, or 360 degrees of the zodiac, the Moon takes only twenty-nine and a half days to make the same journey. If, for example, you are an Aquarius, yet have three other planets in Capricorn, you may actually have more Capricornian characteristics than those of an Aquarius.*

KEYWORDS OF THE SIGNS AND PLANETS

Table 1.2 conveys the keywords of each planet and sign. If your Sun, which represents basic vitality, health, and personality, is placed in Capricorn, you will more than likely be disciplined, structured, and calculating in your climb to the top. If your Moon is in that sign, your emotions, colored by Capricornian traits, will be reserved. Mercury in Capricorn endows a disciplined mind and reticent speech. Venus in Capricorn suggests you are loyal and dependable in love but tend to withhold feelings, while Mars in Capricorn bestows ambition and a tendency toward workaholism, which will help you ascend the ladder of success. Very simply stated, you apply the attributes of a particular sign to qualities represented by the occupying planet. If several planets in your chart inhabit a sign other than that of your Sun, you may find that you identify more with that sign's description. If this is the case, the delineation for both your Sun sign *and* the sign representing the other planets may apply.

---

* An ephemeris, which can be obtained in most bookstores, lists the daily positions of the planets in their zodiacal signs. If you would like a more precise horoscope, which includes the precise sign and degree of your ascendant and the planets, and do not own an astrological software program, the Appendix lists where you can obtain a copy of your horoscope either by mail order or on the web.

Table 1.2 • Keywords of the Planets and Signs

PLANETS	KEYWORDS
Sun	*vitality, individuality, ego*
Moon	*emotions, habits, conditioning*
Mercury	*communication, intelligence*
Venus	*love, beauty, creativity*
Mars	*physical energy, aggression, courage*
Jupiter	*expansion, abundance*
Saturn	*limitation, disciplined, fear*
Uranus	*originality, independent, rebellious*
Neptune	*spiritual, immaterial, imagination*
Pluto	*intensity, power*

SIGNS	KEYWORDS
Aries	*forthright, adventurous, impatient, aggressive*
Taurus	*practical, stable, sensual, stubborn*
Gemini	*talkative, clever, restless, versatile*
Cancer	*emotional, protective, evasive, controlling*
Leo	*proud, ostentatious, creative, dramatic*
Virgo	*analytical, dependable, service-oriented, critical*
Libra	*aesthetic, aloof, harmonious, fair-minded*
Scorpio	*passionate, intense, destructive, relentless*
Sagittarius	*idealistic, arrogant, optimistic, philosophical*
Capricorn	*ambitious, persevering, structured, intolerant*
Aquarius	*social, eccentric, high-strung, objective*
Pisces	*gentle, sensitive, imaginative, addictive*

Your Rising Sign

Since the planets move at a relatively slow pace throughout the day, it is the precise time and place of birth which distinguishes you from someone born on the same day at the other end of the globe. When your horoscope, or picture of the sky at the moment of birth, is translated into a two-dimensional diagram, it is constructed as a circle divided into twelve sectors representing the zodiacal signs. In order to personalize the chart, a line is drawn across the circle representing the horizon where the sky and sea meet. The zodiacal sign appearing on the eastern horizon at the precise moment of birth is called the rising sign, or ascendant. The easternmost point, which signifies the exact time of sunrise, is called the rising, or ascending degree.

If you were born on June 3 at 5:30 A.M. in New York City, Gemini, which the Sun passes through between May 21 and June 20, would be your rising sign as well as your Sun sign since the Sun would just be appearing on the horizon (Fig. 1.2). On the other hand, if you were born on the same day around midday, your Gemini Sun would be directly overhead, situated at the most elevated point in the diagram. This point is known as the midheaven, or MC. With Gemini in this position, the sign in the east would be Virgo. Thus, Gemini would be the Sun sign and Virgo the rising sign (Fig. 1.3). When the Gemini Sun is about to set, it would lie on the descendant, the point diametrically opposed to the ascendant, which would be Sagittarius, the sign 180 degrees from Gemini and the place of sunrise (Fig. 1.4). And at some time between midnight and 1:00 A.M. (on this particular day it is 0:58 A.M.), the Gemini Sun would be at the lowest point in the sky (known as the nadir), and the ascendant, or sign appearing on the horizon, would be Aquarius (Fig. 1.5). Following the above rules, if you know your birth time, it is easy

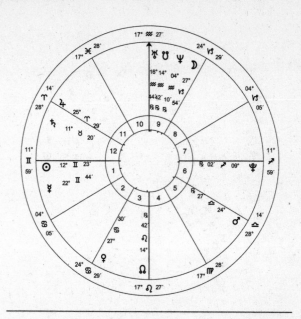

FIGURE I.2 SUNRISE NATAL CHART

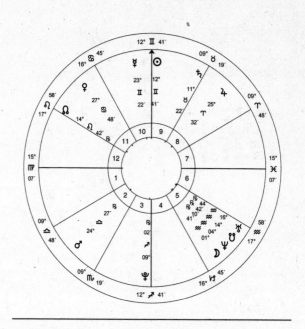

FIGURE I.3 MIDDAY NATAL CHART

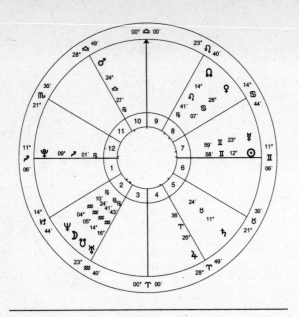

FIGURE I.4 SUNSET NATAL CHART

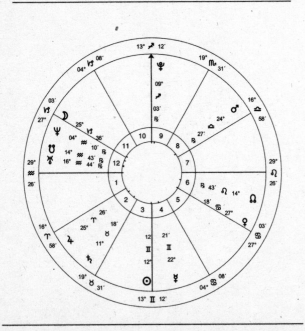

FIGURE I.5 MIDNIGHT NATAL CHART

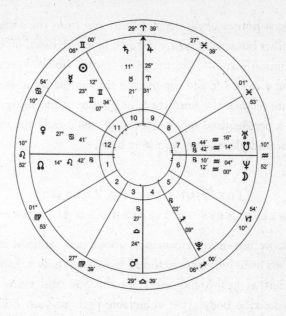

FIGURE 1.6 10:00 A.M. CHART

to approximate in which area of the chart your Sun would be placed. If you were born at 10:00 A.M., for example, your Sun would lie in between the ascendant (position of sunrise) and the midheaven (the position of midday). (See Fig. 1.6.) You may even be able to guess your ascending sign, though to be certain refer to the tables in Appendix I.

After the ascendant is calculated, the planets are placed in their proper zodiacal signs around the chart presenting a two-dimensional view of how the sky appeared at the precise moment of birth as seen from the earth. All the planets will fall either above or below the horizon line. The horoscope is then divided into twelve houses, or arbitrary sectors, with the ascending degree commencing the first house. Some systems employ twelve equilateral houses of 30 degrees measured from the ascendant, while other house systems are unequal in length based on certain astronomical factors. Like the planets, each house represents a different area of life and, by placing the luminaries in their appropriate sectors, the horoscope, or picture of the heavens, becomes a personalized representation of not merely the day but the time and place where you were born.

THE SIGNS OF THE ZODIAC: TWELVE KEYS TO HEALTH AND HAPPINESS

Discovering more information about each zodiacal sign allows us to fully understand all facets of ourselves. Especially significant as health indicators are the Sun and rising signs, which describe body type, vulnerable parts of your body, ailments to which you are prone, and remedies which may prevent, improve, or reverse the situation (Table 1.3).

Each sign of the zodiac is categorized according to its element—fire, earth, air, or water—and its modality, or temperament—cardinal, fixed, or mutable—and derives its attributes, in part, from these categories. (See Table 1.1.) The element describes the sign's essence and how it operates. The modality focuses on one's temperament and mode of expression. Viewing your Sun sign or rising sign in terms of its element and modality will enable you to assess your mental and physical health. These qualities (the elements and modalities) will impart important information regarding each sign's susceptibility to certain ailments as well as its recuperative and healing abilities.

Because the zodiac is divided into four groups of three elements, these divisions are known as the triplicities as follows: fire signs—Aries, Leo, and Sagittarius; earth signs—Taurus, Virgo,

Table 1.3 ◆ Body Parts Ruled by Planets and Signs

PLANETS	BODY PARTS
Sun	*heart, general vitality*
Moon	*breasts, lymphatic system*
Mercury	*nervous system*
Venus	*skin, eyes*
Mars	*level of strength, muscular system, blood*
Jupiter	*healing ability, growths, liver*
Saturn	*skeletal system, joints*
Uranus	*nervous system*
Neptune	*circulatory system*
Pluto	*sexual organs, reproductive system*

SIGNS	BODY PARTS
Aries	*head, face, eyes, nose, ears*
Taurus	*neck, glands*
Gemini	*shoulders, lungs, arms*
Cancer	*breasts, chest, stomach*
Leo	*heart, spine*
Virgo	*intestines, spleen*
Libra	*kidneys, abdomen, pancreas*
Scorpio	*colon, prostate, reproductive organs*
Sagittarius	*hips, thighs, liver, gall bladder*
Capricorn	*knees, teeth, skeletal system*
Aquarius	*ankles, shins*
Pisces	*circulation, feet, lymphatic system*

and Capricorn; air signs—Gemini, Libra, and Aquarius; and water signs—Cancer, Scorpio, and Pisces.

The quadruplicities consist of three groups of four modalities as follows: cardinal signs—Aries, Cancer, Libra, and Capricorn; fixed signs—Taurus, Leo, Scorpio, and Aquarius; mutable signs—Gemini, Virgo, Sagittarius, and Pisces.

ELEMENTS—FIRE, EARTH, AIR, WATER

FIRE SIGNS

Aries, Leo, and Sagittarius are characterized by their vitality, constant physical activity, and the need to burn brightly so their presence is known. They are outgoing, energetic, and do not tolerate idleness even for one moment. While the modality distinguishes the fire signs from one another, each is in danger of potential burnout since they do not permit themselves needed relaxation periods to balance out the extroversion. Driven by an abundance of enthusiasm, vigor, and a strong constitution, fire signs appear to have boundless energy and the ability to sustain themselves on little sleep. At other times, their overpowering zeal can result in a crash and, ultimately, complete exhaustion. Fire signs must learn to pace themselves as many of their ailments are often brought on by the inability to balance overwork and potential fatigue with rest and relaxation.

EARTH SIGNS

Taurus, Virgo, and Capricorns are practical, slow, productive, yet utterly dependable and materialistic. If you want a job done correctly, efficiently, and on time, rely on the persistence of an earth sign to see that project to fruition. Whereas fire signs are impulsive and dislike being burdened by details, earth signs strive for quality and perfection regardless of the amount of time expended. Unlike fire signs, they are not so much concerned with asserting themselves as they are with simply getting the job done. Earth signs are often content to remain in the background and behind the scenes, allowing the fruit of their labor to speak for itself. Multitalented and methodical, once they define their goals and set a course of action, it's full steam ahead. On a physical level, earth signs are the steadiest, strongest, and, as a rule, most resistant to illness due to an amazing stamina. Rooted and stable, they find it very difficult to change deep-set patterns and habits unless they become ill or, at worst, temporarily incapacitated. They are then forced to alter their ways. If, however, a Taurus, Virgo, or Capricorn is prevented from working and earning an income, that's all the incentive he or she will need to adjust his or her lifestyle.

AIR SIGNS

Gemini, Libra, and Aquarius are primarily concerned with the communication and transmission of ideas. Information junkies, media enthusiasts, and excellent conversationalists, air signs can never get enough of the written and spoken word. Their basic motivation is socializing, and they are happiest among friends, colleagues, and intellectual counterparts. In fact, they will do almost anything to avoid being alone. Charming and entertaining, the air signs are consumed with the world of ideas and relationships to the extent that they can easily neglect their health. In fact, they would rather not have to think about physical limitations or even ponder life's practical considerations. Yet, by appealing to both their intellect and reasoning abilities, air signs will eventually respond to their health needs. Once they research and realize the ramifications of unhealthy living for themselves, Geminis, Librans, and Aquarians will take responsibility for their actions.

WATER SIGNS

Cancer, Scorpio, and Pisces, the water signs, are emotional, intuitive, and spontaneous, and rarely take the time to plan, analyze, and reflect upon their actions. Ruled by their feelings, water signs yearn to be cared for and loved, and will quite willingly give in return. Their desire to feel good extends to an attraction to pleasurable, sensual activities from dancing to drinking to sex. As a result, they have practically no tolerance for pain and an enormous difficulty coping with obstacles. Creative, artistic, and generally compassionate, water signs expend so much energy fantasizing about goals they wish to accomplish, little time remains for actively pursuing and attaining them. Due to a proclivity for indulgence and, worst, addictive habits, they must learn to be less reactive, improve objectivity, and employ techniques to strengthen their mental resolve. If an emotional crisis ensues, water signs may automatically eat or drink too much in order to self-medicate and subdue the pain. It is not unusual for Cancerians, Scorpios, and Pisceans to be overweight, suffer from eating disorders, drink too much, or become addicted to drugs. Emotionally sensitive and physically vulnerable, water signs catch cold easily, are prone to allergies, and, as their element indicates, retain fluids.

MODALITIES—CARDINAL, FIXED, AND MUTABLE

CARDINAL SIGNS

If you are an Aries, Cancer, Libra, or Capricorn, you were probably the first one in your class to raise your hand or volunteer for extracurricular activities. Cardinal signs are outgoing, impulsive self-starters who are easily frustrated yet struggle to carry things through to their logical conclusions. Craving constant stimulation, they embark on projects with great enthusiasm and intensity, only to abandon them in midstream due to boredom and waning interest. Applying these qualities to their health, cardinal signs become ill suddenly but recuperate just as quickly. While their ailments are often related to overwork, their disdain for being bedridden or dependent will usually motivate a speedy recovery. They may, however, be too impatient to investigate preventative measures or natural remedies, but instead depend on traditional medicine in a desire to recover quickly.

While each cardinal sign possesses these qualities, the mode of expression differs depending on the sign's element. Aries is the most headstrong of the fire signs, Cancer the most initiating of the water signs, Libra the most forthright of the relationship-oriented air signs, and Capricorn the most enterprising earth sign.

FIXED SIGNS

Fixed signs tend to be stubborn, intractable, determined, and have the ability to exert an enormous amount of willpower and self-control. If your Sun sign is Taurus, Leo, Scorpio, or Aquarius, you relish maintaining autonomy over your life. Once given respect and the authority to make decisions, you will extend the same consideration to those you love. Fixed signs are, as a rule, the most robust and, as a result, the most resistant to disease. However, since they are least apt to alter their lifestyle choices or patterns, they are also most likely to be plagued by chronic ailments. When they finally do become fed up with lingering, annoying symptoms or when they feel they are losing control over their bodies, fixed signs will finally admit that they are due for a change—no matter how difficult that admittance may be.

Taurus is the most stable, rooted, and habitual of the earth signs, Leo the most dictatorial and focused of the fire signs, Scorpio the most obstinate and emotionally controlled of the water signs, and Aquarius the most moody and inflexible of the air signs.

MUTABLE SIGNS

Of all the modalities, mutable signs are the most flexible, easy-going, and changeable. Geminis, Virgos, Sagittarians, and Pisceans share a sense of humility and an almost compulsive need to serve others. While each mutable sign may be the least focused of its particular element, it is also the most malleable, friendly, and willing to adapt to new circumstances. As a rule, mutable signs do not have strong nervous systems and are vulnerable to illness. By the same token, they are more likely to alter their habits and turn to alternative remedies and diverse approaches to improve their health.

Of the air signs, Gemini is the most versatile, moody, and open-minded, while Virgo is the most sensitive, introverted, and self-conscious of the earth signs. Sagittarius, the most self-indulgent fire sign, directs energy toward international adventure and higher knowledge. Pisces is the most emotional, pliable, and insecure of the water signs, and, as such, the least disciplined and persevering.

CONTROL YOUR PHYSICAL DESTINY
THROUGH SELF-UNDERSTANDING

Derived from the combined qualities of its element and modality, your sign's character traits, psychological attributes, and behavior patterns predispose you to certain vulnerabilities and ailments. Since Taureans tend to overeat, they are prone to disorders such as diabetes and hypoglycemia which are exacerbated, if not caused, by dietary imbalances. An awareness of susceptibility may not eradicate these tendencies altogether, but eating healthy, well-balanced meals and following a regular exercise regime can surely "head them off at the pass."

Since Aries rules the head, it is logical to deduce (without even knowing Aries' characteristics) that this sign is impulsive and headstrong. As a result of rushing headfirst, Aries can be accident prone. If you are cognizant of this propensity, it would be wise to slow down and "look before you leap."

More important, each zodiacal sign corresponds to a part of the anatomy, making you susceptible to complaints associated with that body part's weakness or malfunction. For example, one of Leo's vulnerable points is the heart. While Leos may not necessarily have more coronary ailments than do other signs, they are fond of eating rich, high-cholesterol foods, which aggravate this condition. Furthermore, proud, arrogant Leos do not believe in their own mortality and, rather than adhere to rules of moderation, which would engender a longer life, they actually take more risks. This is, of course, ironic since Leos love life more than any other sign.

PLANETS RULE THE SIGNS AND
INFLUENCE YOUR BODY

Each zodiacal sign is also ruled by a planet, whose qualities are shared by that sign. (See Table 1.1.) Just as each zodiacal sign corresponds to a body part or organ, making you vulnerable to ailments related to that sign, the planets do the same. Consequently, the planet ruling the sign of your Sun or ascendant will also alert you to certain weaknesses. Suppose you are a Libra, that is, born between September 23 and October 24, when the Sun traverses the sign of Libra. Since Venus rules Libra, your birth sign, the parts of the body ruled by Libra (kidneys) *and* Venus (eyes, skin) will be sensitive. (See Table 1.3.) If Aries is your ascendant, then Mars is considered to be your ruling planet. In addition to the head and face, which Aries rules, the muscles and blood, which come under the auspices of Mars, can also be weak and/or vulnerable.

NIPPING ILLNESS IN THE BUD
ACCORDING TO YOUR SIGN

By determining which parts of the body are weak or more prone to illness, it is possible to explore ways to strengthen these organs through behavior modification techniques which appeal to each sign's psychological makeup. This procedure may prevent the onset of illness rather than treat it after it has already begun. Evaluating your strengths, weaknesses, and the maladies to which you may be sensitive allows you to ascertain if and how you can alter your lifestyle.

Classifying each sign according to its corresponding herbs, vitamins, Ayurvedic body types, etc., is another way your horoscope can discern which food, physical activities, and remedies are suitable. If, for instance, you wish to embark on an Ayurvedic diet to attain emotional and physical well-being, analyze the *dosha,* or temperament, related to your sign and apply the diet plan associated with that dosha. Although most people are a combination of one or more doshas, your Sun sign is usually a good indicator of body type. (See Appendix II.) It is important to note that the descriptions accompanying each sign are quite general, and an Ayurvedic physician will always thoroughly investigate your entire emotional and physical makeup—which goes beyond Sun sign alone.

In the course of reading this book, you may discover that you identify with the description of a sign other than your Sun or rising sign. For example, your Sun or ascendant may be in Aries, but you could have several planets in Taurus. In addition, Venus, the planet ruling Taurus, may be situated prominently in the horoscope. Unless you have had an in-depth horoscope interpretation, you will be unaware of the details of your chart except for the Sun sign. By all means, take advantage of the suggestions contained in any chapter which may present a more fitting description, since you could have planets positioned in that sign. If you find, for instance, that you identify with Virgo characteristics, follow the dietary suggestions recommended for Virgo even if you have never been troubled by ulcers or intestinal problems—Virgoan ailments. Additionally, certain exercises and remedies may apply to more than one sign. For example, Leo rules the spine, Libra rules the lower back, and Sagittarius rules the sciatic nerve. Many stretches and yoga positions, or asanas, will strengthen each of these areas of the body.

Regardless of your Sun sign, certain recommendations, such as maintaining a proper balance of nutrients and exercising regularly, will improve everyone's general condition. If you are an Aries, for instance, you may be constantly on the go and able to burn up calories effortlessly. It does not, however, mean that you should clog your arteries with fatty food. No matter what your sign, nipping illness in the bud is proof that an ounce of prevention is worth a pound of cure.

The following chapters will describe the physical and psychological attributes associated with each zodiacal sign, accompanied by particular healing techniques which will be most beneficial to those signs. Pay special attention to your Sun sign and your rising sign.* If, for instance, your Sun sign and ascendant belong to the same element or modality, you can be assured

---

* *Appendix I explains how you can determine your ascendant, or rising sign. To be absolutely certain, order a copy of your chart.*

that the description of that sign will be most relevant. It may also overemphasize behavior patterns represented by that sign. Additionally, if a planet is prominently placed on one of the angles in your chart, the sign which that planet rules is vital in determining your own emotional and physical condition.

Chapter 2

Aries the Ram

The Overachiever
Who Forgets to Rest

ARIES THE RAM (MARCH 21–APRIL 19)
RULING PLANET: Mars
ELEMENT: Fire
MODALITY: Cardinal

Positive Aries traits and concepts are pioneering, ambitious, assertive, energetic, independent, enthusiastic, leadership, vitality, daring, innovative, inspirational, willpower, enterprising, exciting, desire, courageous, and passionate.

Negative Aries traits and concepts are selfish, rash, aggressive, angry, greedy, abrasive, reckless, impulsive, insensitive, egocentric, impatient, easily bored, leaves things unfinished, short attention span, temperamental, and childlike.

Parts of the body ruled by Aries include the eyes, head, nose, mouth, ears, forehead, and brain. Its ruling planet, Mars, governs the blood, muscles, and the adrenal glands.

Ailments include fevers, chills, colds, headaches, migraine, earaches, poor eyesight, dental problems, nosebleeds, hyperactivity, and sinus troubles and related allergies, which may cause sneezing and stuffiness.

Professions which display Arian traits of initiative, courage, physical activity and/or excitement include surgeon, doctor, actress, dancer, carpenter, professional athlete, military personnel, hunter, welder, and entrepreneur.

ARIES THE RAM: IMPATIENT AND AGGRESSIVE YET DARING AND INNOVATIVE

The first sign of the zodiac, Aries the Ram is impulsive, impatient, yet wildly creative with unending zest and enthusiasm for everything you experience. Like your symbol, the butting ram that leads with its horns, you act first and think later. Outspoken and eloquent, yet abrasive and candid, you often regret your outbursts moments after they have poured out of your mouth. You believe in being truthful but find it difficult balancing forthrightness with sensitivity, especially in the heat of a passionate argument or difference of opinion. At times, you are too self-centered to see past your own needs and empathize with others. But once you realize that your remarks have been cutting, you immediately accept responsibility for your actions, apologize, and swear you have learned from your mistakes. Unfortunately, you usually do not. Your saving grace is the fact that you are fun-loving, generous, and a great friend, so your sudden surges of enthusiasm and bluntness are often forgiven. You don't dwell on the past, rarely have regrets, and move upward and onward right to the finish line.

High-spirited, passionate, and physically active, Aries, a cardinal fire sign, is never content unless there is a new challenge on the horizon. More interested in the excitement of the game than mastery of it, you often lose interest long before your goals have been attained. If you should emerge victorious, you're off and running to the next activity, hardly taking time to enjoy the fruits of your accomplishments. You view life as a series of challenges to be tackled, contests in which to compete, and battles to be won. Your love of physical activity and desire to excel extends to competitive sports and adventurous activities such as mountain climbing, while your tempestuous and passionate nature provides a strong sexual appetite which never seems to be sated. Completely spontaneous, you often take risks and seek thrills just for the sake of the accompanying adrenaline rush. Your life may be exciting, but it can lead to reckless and careless behavior.

Aries may be innovative, brilliant, and, at times, purely inspirational, but you often overlook the important details. Since one foot is already in the door of the next project before the present one has been brought to fruition, you are always in a time trap, functioning under enormous stress. Though it might appear that Arians find it challenging working under pressure, in actuality, the physical discomfort and mental anxiety which often accompany your lifestyle choices eventually take their toll. You may follow your heart but run the risk of burning out long before the task has been completed. If you take time to relax and smell the roses, even the most mundane task will seem interesting and command your attention.

Don't ever allow yourself to become too depressed. When disappointments materialize, simply chalk them up to experience and get on with your life. Do not leave projects and personal relationships hanging in midstream. Start the day with an early morning run, keep the exercise bicycle within reach, and be sure to join a gym close to the office. Physical release is vital for transforming aggression and hostility into assertiveness and creativity.

PHYSIOGNOMY AND BODY TYPE

Aries usually stands taller than average, is willowy yet amply proportioned, and has well-defined features—high cheekbones, deep-set eyes in a pronounced forehead, an extended chin, and a firm mouth. An active metabolism and addiction to physical exercise will help you shed any unwanted pounds should there be an occasional weight gain. Fasting for two to three days will also bring quick results and satisfy your impatience.* It is important to remember that, if you are over forty, reducing your caloric intake alone just won't do. Unless you follow a vigorous exercise regime several times a week in addition to caloric reduction, you may just have to accept the fact that your midriff bulge and paunchy stomach are here to stay. If, however, you combine diet with exercise, you may be able to meet this challenge head-on.

With Aries ruling the brain, head, and face, you may be prone to fevers, chills, colds, headaches, earaches, poor eyesight, or other ailments affecting those areas. Aries complaints also include dental problems, nosebleeds, hyperactivity, sinusitis, and related allergies, which may cause sneezing and stuffiness.

Your ruling planet, Mars, provides you with deftness and dexterity since it governs the muscles, blood, and circulatory system.

---

* If you have a heart condition, hypertension, or other chronic ailment, consult your doctor before fasting.

Muscle cramps which may plague you from time to time can be eased by a hot bath with appropriate aromatherapy oils in order to relax you and circulate your energy. The rulership of Mars over the adrenal glands explains the lack of impulse control, which leads you to rush headfirst into everything, earning the reputation of being clumsy, careless, and even accident-prone. To avoid a lifetime of cuts, burns, and bruises, slow down, concentrate on what you're doing, and heed the stop signs.

It's important that a traditional first-aid kit always be on hand, as well as alternative remedies which can be immediately applied in case of bodily trauma. Bach Flower Rescue Remedy, the perfect antidote for emotional stress or physical trauma, consists of five flower essences and is available in cream or homeopathic tincture. If you are in an accident or experience cuts or burns, applying Rescue Remedy may prevent your body from plunging into a state of shock. Many people believe that shock, a condition during which the blood pressure is greatly reduced, only arises from a major accident or trauma. In reality, any jolt to the system ranging from a tooth extraction to a burn can propel the body into a mild shock state because the system is adverse to sudden change. Swallowing a few droplets of Rescue Remedy by placing them on your tongue can ease the aftereffects of any trauma. If you have a burn or insect bite, applying the Rescue Remedy or Rescue Cream topically will soothe the pain and hasten the healing process.

HEADACHES AND MIGRAINE

Due to Aries' rulership over the head and face, you are probably no stranger to tension headaches or, worse, the dreaded migraine. While the majority of headaches stem from muscle tension, stress, thinking too much, bad lighting, eyestrain, or skipping meals, which lowers blood sugar and potassium levels, studies have traced the cause of severe headache and other types of chronic pain to the body's inability to produce endorphins—natural painkilling neuropeptides which provide a feeling of well-being.

In addition to reaching into the medicine cabinet for aspirin, or raising the endorphin level through vigorous exercise, there are many remedies which may provide headache relief. If your headache is caused by a low potassium level, replenishing your potassium by taking mineral tablets, eating a banana, or drinking a glass of orange juice is sometimes all you need. Other foods rich in potassium include sweet corn, oranges, bananas, grapefruit, peaches, pineapples, plums, apricots, pears, green beans, turnips, collard greens, brussels sprouts, cauliflower, kale, lettuce, watercress, asparagus, carrots, and celery. Even if the headache is not the result of low potassium, eating these fruits and vegetables is an excellent way to keep potassium levels up. Food which should be avoided include processed foods and delicatessen meats (including hot dogs), which contain sodium nitrite and other food preservatives and additives. Monosodium glutamate (MSG), a preservative contained in meat tenderizer and a staple of Chinese cooking, is notorious for producing headaches and even severe allergic reactions. Many restaurants no longer use MSG or will, upon request, prepare your food without it.

In addition to lack of potassium (obtained from the above-mentioned foods) and calcium (supplied by dairy products and leafy greens), certain headaches may be the result of niacin, iron, and pantothenic acid deficiencies. In fact, B-complex vitamins, contained in yeast, breads, cereal, etc., strengthen the nerves and ease the tension that is sometimes responsible for headaches. It is recommended that you start the morning with a heaping tablespoon of brewer's yeast, one of the best sources of vitamin B. Camouflage its taste by mixing it in your cereal or yogurt and adding fruit and/or honey. You will forget that the brewer's yeast, which when taken alone has an awful aftertaste, is part of this mixture. (See Appendix II for which foods contain particular nutrients.)

Tension headaches may also be the result of premenstrual syndrome (PMS), in the case of women, or depression, which sets in during times of inactivity. Aries should never be cooped up for too long, and often the antidote for a tension headache is fresh air and plenty of exercise.

Experts are still in the dark as to why headaches occur and research continues to discover how to treat and, ultimately, prevent their onset. It is important to avoid stressful situations and to relax the upper part of the body, especially the head and neck. Mild head and neck tension may be relieved each morning by the following simple head and neck rolls:

1. Stand erect or sit in an upright chair with your back completely straight.
2. Lower and relax your head so that your chin is resting on your chest.
3. Moving counterclockwise, roll your head in a circular motion very slowly. First, move it as far to the right as you can so that you can see behind your right shoulder, as far back so that you can see the ceiling, as far to the left so you can see behind your left shoulder, and then back to center, where it once again touches your chest.
4. Repeat the same exercise but begin in a clockwise motion. Move your head as far to the left as you can so that you can see behind your left shoulder, as far back so that you can see

the ceiling, as far to the right so you can see behind your right shoulder, and then back to center, where it once again touches your chest.

5. Repeat each movement five times, alternating so that you begin by turning counterclockwise, then clockwise, counterclockwise, clockwise, as slowly as possible so that at each juncture (right shoulder, back of the head, and left shoulder) you stop for a few seconds.

Another exercise simply involves moving your head up and down and left to right to stretch the neck muscles, which, in turn, will relax your face and head.

The following exercises repeated ten times will soothe the muscles of the face and the head, and may relieve headache suffering.

1. Lift eyebrows up quickly, relax, and let them drop.
2. Squint eyes and release.
3. Lift your right eyebrow up, pause, and release.
4. Lift your left eyebrow up, pause, and release.
5. Yawn wide and close.
6. Open and stretch your mouth widely as if you are ready to scream. Slowly close.
7. Wrinkle and squeeze nose upward, as if smelling a foul odor.
8. Make faces.

To reduce pain, first try massaging the temples by applying acupressure with the thumb and forefinger. Thereafter, use both thumbs to apply pressure to the bony ridges at the back of the neck.

If your headache persists, occurs more frequently, and/or is accompanied by other symptoms such as nausea, dizziness, blurred vision, or numbness, see a doctor immediately.

Whereas a headache may incapacitate you only briefly, as it quickly responds to aspirin, a migraine may last anywhere from a few hours to a few days and can be completely debilitating to the point that the sufferer's only escape is sleep. Migraines are characterized by intensely throbbing pain on one or both sides of the head and may be accompanied by nausea, vomiting, dizziness, and tremors. There are many theories as to why migraines occur, but none has been proven. Since these headaches are aggravated by tension or stress, try the aforementioned headache remedies and general relaxation exercises as an attempt to control excruciating pain.

Because it can help detect certain physical changes before they actually occur, biofeedback may help migraine sufferers to recognize the first sign that these dreadful headaches are approaching. Consequently, certain stress-reduction techniques such as yoga, meditation, and tai chi may bring some relief although not alleviate the symptoms altogether. Elimination of certain foods from the diet may also prevent and, at times, control the onset of migraine and other vascular headaches.

Outdoor activities that provide Aries natives with fresh air and cold wind on their faces such as mountain climbing, hiking, swimming, and vigorous walking may assuage stress, thus reducing migraine severity and frequency. If you are in the throes of a spell, temporary relief may be obtained by using cold packs or pressing on the bulging artery found in front of the ear on the painful side of the head. Unfortunately, none of these alternatives is a cure. Although strong medication has recently been developed to combat these debilitating headaches, there is presently no miracle drug which completely relieves the agony.

COLDS AND FEVERS

With the head in command, Arians are also prone to colds, fevers, and sinusitis. Fevers are not considered to be illnesses as such but are rather a line of defense against illness. Since you perspire profusely when you are feverish, it is important to replenish bodily fluids by drinking plenty of liquids—water, beet juice, carrot juice, and herbal teas are recommended. Chamomile tea reduces inflammation, linden tea promotes sweating, and willow bark contains salicylate (the active ingredient which gives aspirin its anti-inflammatory power). If you cannot tolerate substances containing aspirin, black elder tea may do the trick. Applying wet compresses to the forehead, wrists, and calves while sucking on an ice cube acts to reduce the body's temperature and allay fever.

Who among us hasn't had a cold? While there are no "official" cures or medications for the common cold, there are remedies which can provide relief for the sneezing, coughing, and wheezing that can sometimes make life temporarily unbearable. Vitamin C taken on a daily basis offers the best prevention and, once you feel a cold coming on, megadoses (2000 milligrams) taken for the short term will probably not cause any problems. It is a good idea, however, to check with your doctor since large doses of vitamin C can have adverse effects. Rich sources of vitamin C include lemons, oranges, grapefruit, cranberries, tomatoes— which can be eaten raw or in juice form—and rose hips taken in powder form or as tea. If you choose to make fresh rose hip tea, be sure to strain the tea thoroughly—like fresh roses, rose hips are enveloped by thorns. In addition to vitamin C, rose hips contain vitamins A, E, B_1, B_2, K, niacin, calcium, phosphorus, and iron.

If all else fails, the healing powers of chicken soup should seriously be considered. Hot chicken soup can unclog mucus in the nasal passages. After all, thousands of Jewish mothers and grandmothers who've prepared and served this piping-hot liquid to children like myself couldn't possibly be wrong!

ECHINACEA AND GOLDENSEAL

In recent years, wild herbs like echinacea and goldenseal have been packaged and promoted as miracle cures for the common cold. Indigenous to North America, these two "magical" herbs have been utilized for centuries by Native Americans to cure sore throats, flus, and colds. In Europe, where homeopathic medicine, herbal cures, spas, and other alternative treatments are much more acceptable than in the United States, a homeopathic tincture of echinacea is often prescribed for swollen glands, scratchy throat, or difficulty swallowing. Named for the seallike scars on its golden-yellow root, goldenseal, which can be sniffed through the nostrils in powder form, clears out the nasal and bronchial passages. Both echinacea and goldenseal are also available in tablet form. Like many other herbs, these two are potent and should not be taken in large doses if you are pregnant, have high blood pressure, or suffer from hypoglycemia. Nor should they be taken for extended periods of time. Spirulina, bee pollen, and royal jelly are also good protein supplements, which strengthen the immune system. Sage, peppermint, and spearmint teas have a soothing effect and may help to shorten the duration of a cold.

Obviously, body aches and fever brought on by a cold may be relieved by over-the-counter remedies such as aspirin or Tylenol. Antihistamines may stop sneezing and help to dry up a runny nose and eyes, and decongestants can unstuff the nose. Be sure to cough and sneeze into tissues that can be easily disposed of, wash your hands often, and try to keep the germs from spreading to family and friends.

With germs most likely to attack a run-down, weak immune system, bed rest is probably, in the end, the best antidote for preventing colds from graduating into more serious ailments such as bronchitis, influenza, and pneumonia. All the vitamin C and echinacea in the world will not prevent colds and flus if the body is tired or completely run down, since the immune system will not be in fighting form. Like any other ailment, if a cold persists longer than a week to ten days, see your physician immediately.

SINUSITIS

Sinusitis results when the sinus cavities around the nose and eyes fail to filter out bacteria. It makes its presence known when nasal passages become inflamed with yellow or green mucus, or when swelling, severe pain, and/or headaches ensue. This condition may be the result of an infection which has traveled from the upper respiratory tract to the membrane lining of the sinus cavities, or the result of an allergic reaction to dust, ragweed, animal hair, and/or smoke.

If you are a chronic sinusitis sufferer, it is important to visit an allergist to see if the problem is allergy induced. If so, it is advisable to keep your house pet-free. An air purifier will help keep each room fresh and clean by removing irritating particles from the air. If you move into a new house, be sure to paint the walls and fumigate the carpets since animal hair, fur, and dander (especially from dogs, cats, and rabbits) linger on even after the pets have gone. In addition, keep your environment smoke-free and be sure to dust regularly and vacuum thoroughly to rid the house of dust mites. (See "Living with Asthma" in Chapter 4.)

Humidity also eases sinusitis. Whenever you feel especially

stuffy, take a hot, steamy shower or stand over a pot of boiling chamomile tea with a towel over your head, forcing the steam directly into the nostrils. A cold-mist vaporizer in the bedroom will help the nasal and sinus passages from drying out and will allow a decent night's sleep. Be careful to keep the apparatus clean since the vaporizer itself is a good breeding place for bacteria.

Rubbing vitamin E oil in your nose will ease swelling or pain. Ingesting vitamin C fights infection, increasing protein intake helps restore damaged sinus tissue, and vitamin A strengthens the mucous membranes in the nose and throat. A saline solution consisting of a teaspoon of salt and a dash of baking soda dissolved in two cups of warm water can be inhaled up each nostril to flush out nasal secretions.

YOGIC BREATHING

Pranayama, or yogic breathing, consists of breathing through the nostrils so that *prana,* Sanskrit for "life's breath," is gathered and utilized to open your nasal passages and purify the system of toxins, which are ingested daily. In his book *Perfect Health,* Deepak Chopra recommends that you should start and end your day with Pranayama, which should take about ten minutes. According to Chopra, begin by sitting with your spine very straight and resting your feet firmly on the floor. Close your eyes and try to rid your mind of all thoughts. Beginning on the exhale and ending on the inhale, exhale and inhale through your left nostril while simultaneously pressing your thumb against the right nostril. Do this by gently closing the right nostril with your thumb and slowly exhaling through your left nostril, then, inhale easily through your left nostril. Alternate by closing your left nostril with your middle and ring finger, and exhaling and inhaling through your right nostril. After five minutes relax your arms at your side, let go of your upright position, and sit comfortably with your eyes closed.[2]

Although decongestant tablets help shrink the blood vessels so air can flow into the nose, do not use these or over-the-counter nasal sprays unless you have the go-ahead from your doctor. While they can initially shrink the nasal lining, they later cause more swelling. If all else fails, see a doctor, who may treat the sinusitis with antibiotics.

Deep breathing will also improve your impulse control. The next time you feel yourself getting flustered, avoid the maelstrom of anger and frustration. Instead, try to relax and practice Pranayamic breathing. After five or ten minutes, you'll have found the needed respite, and become energized and ready to return to work.

MINERAL SALT

The human body contains twelve essential biochemical mineral salts which are constantly depleted and replenished by the food we eat. Each salt is associated with the zodiacal sign whose corresponding body part or organ reaps its benefits. Potassium phosphate (Kali. phos.), the tissue salt associated with Aries, prevents nervousness, insomnia, skin rashes, and alleviates headaches, especially those which stem from lack of potassium. Foods rich in potassium phosphate include potatoes, green vegetables, onions, walnuts, oranges, tomatoes, lemons, pineapples, apples, raisins, and milk.

AYURVEDA

While most people are not pure Ayurvedic types, Aries, a cardinal fire sign, fits the profile of the Pitta personality, whom Deepak Chopra, in his book *Perfect Health,* describes as being short-tempered, liking challenges, reacting rashly and irritably under stress, having a keen mind, and possessing physical strength. Impulsive, rash behavior and a fiery temperament may give way to skin rashes, fevers, and inflammations. It is important to provide balance and moderation through coolness, attention to leisure, exposure to natural beauty, decreased stimulants, and, most important, rest and relaxation. When you are feeling serene, your negative emotions will be expressed through activity rather than aggression.

You are naturally impatient by nature and your eating habits are therefore no different. If your blood-sugar level drops and calls out for food, you will abide without taking the time to prepare a healthy meal. Unlike other signs, you do not view cuisine preparation as an art; you see food merely as necessary fuel. You have no desire to spend a great deal of time cooking and will gobble down whatever is available. To avoid unhealthy eating habits, keep fresh fruit and vegetable salad in the refrigerator at all times. This works perfectly, according to Ayurveda, which promotes cool and bitter foods such as bitter greens, chicory, endive, radicchio, and romaine lettuce to Pitta types. High-fiber vegetables and grains are recommended, and drinking tonic water before meals is also advisable. Do not eat sour foods like pickles, yogurt, vinegar, sour cream, and cheese, or anything fermented, like old cheese or alcohol. Breakfast should consist of cold cereal, cinnamon toast, and apple juice. Astringent spices like cardamom, cilantro (green coriander leaves), cinnamon, coriander (seeds), dill, fennel, mint, saffron, and turmeric are good. Ginger is an all-around remedy and can be used in tea and in cooking. Asian cuisine, which utilizes ginger and many other Pitta spices, is highly recommended.

Pitta types are generally overheated, and as such you are more comfortable in a cold and windy climate to subdue the natural heat you generate. Strenuous and invigorating outdoor physical activity like mountain climbing, skiing, brisk walking, jogging, hiking, and swimming suits you perfectly. Weight lifting, aerobics, and competitive sports may also appeal to you though you must watch your impatience, short temper, and tendency to take the game you are playing too much to heart. Try abiding by the adage which suggests that it is not important if you win or lose but how you play the game that counts. Risk taking and a love of speed could lead you to race-car driving, bunjee jumping, skydiving, and other satisfying, thrill-seeking (and perhaps dangerous) activities. Just be certain that you "play against type" and exert utmost caution and impeccable judgment. Since your mind works as quickly as your body, mental exercise such as voracious reading and research will also be appealing.

HERBS AND SPICES

The following herbs and spices can be used as condiments or in tea form. Basil is an aromatic herb used in cooking and for healing wounds. Tea made from borage, a common garden herb containing potassium, calms nerves and is highly recommended for lowering fever and reducing inflammation and swelling. Comfrey tea prevents colds and, if applied externally, can soothe insect bites and bruises or be used as a compress for eye injuries and sties. Cayenne powder, a very hot spice contained in red powder form, is a great stimulant and body purifier. While it can prevent colds, it will cause reddening of the skin if used to excess. Garlic, an all-round healer, fights infections and colds. It can be used in cooking, eaten raw, or taken in capsule form once a day. Other Aries herbs include bergamot for mental relaxation; elderberry for lowering fevers and soothing

burns; thyme for abating fever, headaches, and migraine; lavender for headaches and migraines; and sassafras, a tasty tea and
blood purifier which may prevent colds. It can also be utilized
as an eyewash for inflammations. Licorice, peppermint, and
spearmint tea are extremely soothing for hyperactive Arians.
Chamomile is an all-round panacea but especially beneficial for
allaying headaches, insomnia, and earaches.

Herbal teas which have a tranquilizing effect are valerian (the
same root as Valium), elderberry, chamomile, comfrey, dandelion (which contains Kali. Phos.), ginseng, licorice, peppermint,
spearmint, and any commercial Sleepy Time teas (whose main
ingredient is chamomile). If taken at the end of the day or before
bedtime, any of these teas will help you unwind and fall asleep.

AROMATHERAPY AND ESSENTIAL OILS

Since Aries are prone to headaches and migraines, certain essential oils can calm your nerves and curb aggression. Rub
twelve drops of lemon, chamomile, juniper, or marjoram oil
onto the solar plexus, the emotional center of the body, or add
to bathwater. A scent both fragrant and personally satisfying such
as jasmine, rose, or orange blossom can work wonders. Sweet and
cool aromas like sandalwood, rose, mint, cinnamon, and jasmine
are wonderful for clearing up the head and sinuses. They can be
burned as incense, used as bath oil, or inhaled through the nostrils. For conjunctivitis and sore eyes, soak cotton pads in a solution of chamomile and boiled water, and place on the eyes after
they have cooled.

Eucalyptus oil is fantastic for treating fevers, sore throat, inflamed nasal membranes, asthma, and the croup. Eucalyptus is
the primary ingredient in many commercial chest rubs, nasal
sprays, and cough and sore-throat lozenges. Inhaling steam

formed when leaves or oil are boiled in water by draping a towel over the head is effective for relieving congestion.

GEM AND COLOR THERAPY

If you were born between March 21 and March 31, your birthstone is the aquamarine, a beautiful blue semiprecious stone. If you were born between April 1 and April 19, your birthstone is the diamond, an expensive white precious stone which is also associated with the planet Venus. The metal ruling Aries is iron, but these gemstones should always be set in gold. The color red is associated with assertive, action-oriented Mars, Aries' ruling planet, and, therefore, stones like coral, bloodstone, carnelian, and ocher will provide energy if you are tired, and courage in times of uncertainty.

Chapter 3

Taurus the Bull

The Key to Joy
Is Learning Moderation

TAURUS THE BULL (APRIL 20–MAY 20)
RULING PLANET: Venus
ELEMENT: Earth
MODALITY: Fixed

Positive Taurus traits and concepts are industrious, reliable, steady, pragmatic, determined, independent, gentle, sensual, serene, creative, musical, tolerant, frugal, affectionate, hospitable, and generous.

Negative Taurus traits and concepts are indolent, obstinate, self-indulgent, extravagant, overeater, wasteful, hot-tempered, dull, greedy, cheap, rigid, excessive, inflexible, possessive, jealous, controlling, materialistic, arrogant, and obsessive.

Parts of the body ruled by Taurus include the throat, neck, lymph glands, thyroid, and lymphatic system. Its ruling planet, Venus, governs the eyes, skin, and the kidneys.

Ailments include obesity, gallstones, diabetes, heart problems, sore throat, swollen lymph glands and nodes, mononucleosis, thyroid irregularity, stiff neck, laryngitis, tonsillitis, and skin rashes.

Professions which exemplify the Taurean affinity with investments, business, creativity, and/or long-term planning include clothing designer, sculptor, nutritionist, singer, artist, landscape gardener, interior designer, architect, horticulturist, economist, investment banker, financier, broker, real estate agent, retailer, and gemologist.

TAURUS THE BULL:
OBSTINACY AND DETERMINATION
KEEP ILLNESS AWAY

The most stubborn, persistent, resourceful, and inflexible sign of the zodiac, Taurus, a fixed earth sign, is consumed with maintaining complete control over life by proceeding slowly and deliberately. A striking combination of the indolent cow and determined bull, you are often infuriated at close friends who constantly goad you to move faster or discontinue a long-term project and start anew. Though you are known to procrastinate, if anyone is determined to fight to the finish it is certainly Taurus the Bull. Unwilling to relinquish anything earned or "acquired," you can be a relentless business person, a possessive, jealous partner (personal and professional), and/or an overprotective, controlling parent. On the other hand, your ruling planet is Venus, named for the Roman goddess of love and beauty, and, as such, you are creative, gentle, loving, and sensual.

Although you are one of the most pragmatic, responsible, and stable signs of the zodiac, your passions, instincts, and sensual appetite can, at times, override sound judgment. Fair-minded and unselfish beyond words, you treasure friendships but, in return, demand exactly what you give—devotion and trust. If, however, you are hurt, slighted, or feel betrayed (though it takes a long time for you to reach that point), the gentle bovine will become a raging bull, and you'll sever the most intimate relationship on the spot, without so much as a backward glance.

Your strong, tough constitution coupled with immense obstinacy and an aversion to dependency prevents you from becoming seriously ill. When under the weather you will avoid going to the doctor or asking for help—even when you are feeling weak or sick. By the same token, if infirmity results, your obsessive self-reliance provides the willpower for a speedy recuperation. Once your mind is made up, lethargy and complacency take a backseat, and the most industrious, productive, and single-minded personality under the Sun emerges.

The placidity and fierce determination that propels you through life, however, often conceals a deep-rooted insecurity which can culminate in an almost obsessive need to be loved. When feeling inadequate, insecure, or confronted with what appears to be insurmountable obstacles, Taureans often sink into depressions from which they do not easily emerge. To allay stress, you tend to seek solace and medicate your pain in the form of promiscuity, overspending, and/or overeating. While you may indeed find temporary gratification, these excessive and indulgent behavior patterns will plague you throughout your entire life, affecting both mental and physical health.

PHYSIOGNOMY AND BODY TYPE

Taureans are often characterized by a moon-shaped face, rosy cheeks, intense stare, pug nose, rigid mouth, extended chin, thick neck, and plump body. Most are short to average in height, built rather solidly, and, more often than not, possess a full-bodied figure. Your sedentary lifestyle and enjoyment of good food makes it that much more difficult to maintain what you perceive should be your ideal weight. You may even view yourself as heavier than you actually are, leading to enormous self-image problems and even more overeating to assuage the emotional pain. In reality, the physical attributes you strive for may be unrealistic in relation to your body structure. Learn to value inner beauty, take pride in your vast accomplishments, and, most important, do not give in to peer pressure by adapting yourself to societal expectations.

CONQUERING THE BATTLE OF THE BULGE

Due to image problems and low self-esteem, which frequently accompany the stigma of being even slightly overweight or anything other than bone thin, you may have, at one time or other, struggled with eating disorders like anorexia or bulimia in the struggle to maintain your "ideal" weight. (Bulimia, characterized by binging and purging, usually aided by laxatives and/or vomiting, and anorexia, a condition marked by a refusal to eat, are symptomatic of the desire to be thin and the need to be in complete control over one's life.) More common among Taureans, however, is chronic overeating. Aside from affecting one's physical and mental well-being, obesity is a contributing factor to kidney malfunction, gallstones, diabetes, heart disease, and certain cancers of the stomach and colon. Some studies even link specific types of breast cancers to a high percentage of body fat.

So, if obesity is detrimental to both mental and physical health, why is it so difficult for Taureans to practice good eating habits and increase physical exercise in order to shed those unwanted pounds? And why do most Taureans spend a lifetime either overweight or yo-yo dieting, that is, losing and gaining weight over and over again?

Aside from genetic predisposition or glandular disorders, one answer may lie in the Taurean need to balance complete autonomy with an overwhelming desire to feel good and be loved. When emotionally stressed, hurt, angry, or sad, food is often used to tranquilize the pain and/or as a reward for enduring a difficult time. Unfortunately, once habitual Taureans fall into poor eating patterns or use food as a substitute for contentment or love, it is a constant uphill battle and an extremely difficult pattern to change.

It is possible to point your obstinacy and determination in the direction of a balanced diet combined with a moderate, steady exercise plan. Looking and feeling better about yourself will give you the self-esteem necessary to pursue more relationships, friendships, job opportunities, and promotions. Habitual, structured Taureans need to follow a prearranged eating plan setting forth precisely which foods should be consumed daily and those which should be eliminated from the diet altogether. A modified, predetermined exercise plan is recommended to suit your slow, deliberate pace and, at the same time, accelerate your metabolism to burn up excessive calories.

EATING MODIFICATION PLANS
WHICH FINALLY WORK

Arduous as it may be, it is imperative that you permanently change your daily habits by eating three healthy, nutritious meals with little snacking, and drinking eight glasses of water. Limit your salt intake and consumption of salty foods, which cause the body to retain water. If you eliminate fatty foods that are both high in calories and cholesterol, and concentrate on protein, fruits, vegetables, and carbohydrates, you will automatically feel lighter and be healthier. The following is a recommended nutritious, well-balanced, and low-calorie daily diet plan* which emphasizes protein, fruits, vegetables, and carbohydrates:

- Eat no more than 8 ounces raw or 6 ounces cooked lean meat, poultry, and fish daily. Trim visible skin and fat. When cooking meat, drain off the fat after cooking. If boiling meat in stews, gravies, soups, or sauces, strain the fat. Broil, bake, or grill rather than fry. Fish can be eaten fresh, frozen, or canned in water (if canned in oil, rinse thoroughly). Greatly limit your intake of tongue, kidneys, sweetbreads, heart, and brains as they are very high in cholesterol. Liver, a good source of iron, is also high in cholesterol, so eat no more than 3 ounces per month.
- One cup serving of cooked beans, peas, or lentils, or 3 ounces of soybean curd (tofu), can replace a 3-ounce serving of meat, poultry, or fish.
- Eat no more than 3 eggs per week.
- Drink 6 to 8 glasses of water daily.

* This is the diet plan recommended by the National Institutes of Health.

- Two cups skim milk or low-fat or nonfat yogurt should be eaten daily.
- Eat 5 or more servings per day of fruits and vegetables, which may include 1 medium-size piece of fruit, $\frac{1}{2}$ cup fruit or vegetable juice, and $\frac{1}{2}$ to 1 cup cooked or raw vegetables. Eat only one serving of a starchy vegetable such as corn, potatoes, lima beans, green peas, winter squash, yams, and sweet potatoes. Olives, avocados, and coconut are all rich in fat and should be eaten sparingly.
- Eat 6 or more servings per day of the following breads, cereals, pasta, and starchy vegetables, each of which are considered to be the equivalent of 1 serving:
  1 slice bread—this includes wheat, rye, raisin, or white bread, English muffins, frankfurter and hamburger buns, water (not egg) bagels, pita bread, tortillas (not fried);
  $\frac{1}{4}$ cup nugget or bud-type cereal, $\frac{1}{2}$ cup hot cereal, or 1 cup flaked cereal;
  1 cup cooked rice or pasta;
  $\frac{1}{4}$ to $\frac{1}{2}$ cup starchy vegetables as mentioned above (only one serving per day should be eaten);
  a few teaspoons of oil and butter.

DIETING TIPS

While it is extremely difficult for Taureans to change their habits, you are still determined, persevering, and stubborn, especially in situations which require great tenacity and resolve. Plan exciting meals, do not skip any of the aforementioned categories, and vary your diet within each food group. In order to make your diet plan interesting, try substituting some low-fat, low-calorie recipes for high-calorie meals. (See Chapter 6.) Remember that if you skip one meal, you may find yourself so hungry that it will lead to binge eating later in the day.

Get into the habit of drinking six to eight glasses of water daily along with other noncaffeinated beverages. Herbal teas especially recommended are aromatic blackberry and elderberry teas. Chicory coffee, an herbal substitute, has a distinct flavor which appeals to many Taureans, who rely on caffeine to get them through the day. Although chicory is noncaffeinated, it may satisfy the psychological urge for coffee. If you own a juicer or blender, you should take the time to make fresh fruit or vegetable juice or skim-milk malteds, which are both nutritious and filling. Although it can be agonizing for Taureans to discard old habits, make up your mind to alter your eating patterns to win the battle of the bulge once and for all.

Luckily, vanity and a fierce determination—if you wish to draw on them—can provide the willpower necessary to change your lifestyle. If you are unable to accomplish this on your own, do not feel embarrassed to see a counselor who specializes in eating disorders, or join a weight loss group such as Weight Watchers or a twelve-step program such as Overeaters Anonymous (OA), which use support systems to aid the dieter. OA provides an opportunity to work with a sponsor—someone you can contact for unconditional support whenever you get the urge to eat. For a nominal fee, Weight Watchers offers encouragement at weekly meetings where you get weighed and hear members talk about diet plans, exercise programs, and permanent lifestyle revisions. This type of group may give you the inspiration you need since you will definitely get your money's worth—especially when the pounds start to drop. While you may not enjoy airing your difficulties, you may just have to admit that struggling in isolation is invariably fruitless.

Other tips include viewing yourself in—rather than avoiding—mirrors and weighing yourself several times a week. If you have never had a weight problem this may seem absurd, but I can assure you that this Taurean has gone through long intervals shunning both mirrors and the scale in order to avoid facing the music. However, once you cannot fit into the previous season's clothes and need an additional notch on your belt, you must face the truth and take the proverbial bull by the horns. When you start to exceed your ideal weight by two to three pounds, nip any weight gain right in the bud. Start at once to reduce your caloric intake and increase daily physical activity. To lose just one pound, you must burn 3,500 calories more than you ingest. Therefore, if you reduce your caloric intake by 500 calories per day or 3,500 calories per week, you will lose one pound weekly. There is a wealth of books on the market which contain calorie counters and various exercise recommendations accompanied by a chart of the calories expended in each.

For those Taureans who are accustomed to feeling completely sated at mealtime, this food plan may seem like very light fare. At first, feeling light and hungry may lead to irritability and moodiness, as though something is missing. Don't lose heart. Instead of reaching for food, indulge in a physical activity which allows the release of pent-up aggression. Walking, dancing, golfing, swimming, running, or bicycling will each do the trick.

Visualization Exercises

Try the following visualization exercise as soon as you wake up in the morning, even before you get out of bed.

1. Sit up straight, close your eyes, and imagine that you are suddenly weightless, floating either in the water or on air.

2. Stay in that position for about five to ten minutes, erasing all other thoughts from your mind.

3. Retaining that feeling of weightlessness and keeping your eyes closed, start imagining what you might look like from head to toe if you could have your ideal physique.

4. Keeping that image in your mind's eye, picture all the things you might be able to accomplish if you were thinner, such as running a mile without getting out of breath, or wearing a particular outfit which you may have outgrown.

If you begin the day by imagining that you are lithe and thin, adjusting your eating habits to suit that feeling may become easier. Once you recognize, and look forward to, the immediate rewards likely to materialize the moment you achieve your weight loss goal, you may be able to internalize these external images, and sweeping changes are bound to occur.

PHYSICAL EXERCISE

It is not enough to change your eating habits without weaving an exercise plan into your daily life, especially if you are over forty and your metabolism must work twice as hard as it once did to burn those extra calories. In addition to burning calories, exercise functions as the supreme appetite suppressant, as it increases one's level of endorphins—chemicals which provide a feeling of well-being and even euphoria. When anxiety and depression have been alleviated, you will feel serene. You will have no need for food to pacify, tranquilize, or fill an empty space. Once you start shedding pounds, your self-esteem will be automatically lifted.

Before you embark on an exercise plan, check with your doctor to see which exercises best suit your age group and physical condition. If you have been inactive for quite some time, begin with lighter movements such as pleasure walking, gardening, yard work, or dancing. More strenuous aerobic exercises such as swimming, jogging, bicycling, or taking brisk walks three to four times a week for at least thirty minutes will condition your heart and lungs as well as burn excess calories. Remember not to force more physical activity than you can handle.

Going to a fitness club at specified times each week may help you establish a routine. Consider buying workout equipment for your home if you are embarrassed to go to a public gym. Finding an exercise partner to prod you along may be just the incentive you need to alter sedentary habits. Since Taureans prefer warmth, winter activities should include swimming and tennis, which can be done indoors and will also help prevent you from catching colds and chills.

REMEDYING THROAT AND NECK PROBLEMS

While it's simple to blame the inability to lose weight on low thyroid function, most Taureans gain weight from overeating, pure and simple, and not exercising enough to counteract the excess calories. Since Taurus governs the thyroid gland, located at the base of the neck, people born under this sign may suffer from an underactive thyroid, resulting in a sluggish metabolism and the inability to burn calories quickly. If you are diagnosed with a thyroid malfunction, it may be caused by lack of iodine.

One of the best sources of iodine is kelp, a variety of seaweed often used as a salt substitute which can be eaten fresh in salads or taken in tablet form. As an added bonus, kelp also contains vitamins B complex, D, E, K, calcium, and magnesium. (See Appendix II—"Vitamins.") Iodine is also readily obtained from fish (especially saltwater and shellfish), iodine supplements, and/or fish oil in capsule form. (I would not personally recommend pure fish oil as the taste is quite unpleasant.) If these do not help, your physician can prescribe medication to regulate the thyroid and restore the proper metabolic rate.

A stiff neck is another common Taurean complaint especially during the winter, when you are vulnerable to wind and chills. When the weight of the world seems to rest on your shoulders, your neck will respond to stress by feeling heavier and remaining in a stationary, uncomfortable position, making it difficult to move it from side to side. To combat rigidity, try the following exercise.

1. Sit or stand with your head held high so that your neck is elongated as much as possible.
2. Slowly, tilt your neck forward as far as it goes. Do not force it to bend any farther than it naturally can move.
3. Slowly, move it backward as far as it goes.
4. Slowly, tilt your head toward one shoulder and then tilt it toward the other shoulder while holding your neck high, keeping your shoulder down.
5. Rotate your neck in place until you feel that some of the kinks have been unknotted.
6. Shake your head aggressively from side to side and front to back.

In addition to this exercise, lightly massage your neck daily, especially beneath the earlobes. If stiffness occurs, apply a heating pad, eucalyptus oil, or a mentholated ointment such as tiger balm (a combination of camphor and menthol), which will draw the heat out.

Feeling ill at ease with their bodies, Taureans often have very poor posture, which can also increase tension and cause pain in the neck and shoulder blades. The Alexander Technique, whereby you imagine yourself to be a beautiful, graceful swan by elongating your neck and improving your posture, will help your body and improve self-esteem. (See Chapter 6.)

Since Taurus rules the neck and throat, it would be a rarity if someone born under the sign of the Bull has not at one time been affected by a stiff neck, frequent sore or scratchy throat, laryngitis, tonsillitis, swollen glands (lymph nodes in the neck beneath the chin), or mononucleosis.

With your ruling planet, Venus, prevailing over the eyes, skin, and kidneys, you may also be prone to nearsightedness, skin rashes, and water retention. Many Taureans are blessed with beautiful singing and speaking voices. But just as the vocal cords are a gift, they are also the Taurean's most vulnerable point. When the flu season approaches, make sure your wardrobe includes hats, scarves, turtleneck sweaters, and mufflers, which prevent the wind from beating down upon your face and neck. Early signs that germs are on the rampage may come in the form of a scratchy throat or swollen glands, which, as the body's first line of defense, become enlarged when they fight infection.

HOME REMEDIES

A sore throat can be extremely painful and may indicate that a cold or flu is not far behind. It may precede a virus or bacteria invasion, or could mean that you have used your voice more than necessary. Throat sprays or lozenges containing either phenol or zinc offer short-term relief. Gargling with chamomile tea is a popular remedy and will be comforting if the soreness is high enough in the throat for the gargle to reach.

Another simple remedy for sore throat or difficulty swallowing is gargling with lukewarm salt water. Diluted lemon juice with or without honey in lukewarm water is also a good home remedy. Since lemons are an all-purpose healer, it doesn't hurt to squeeze lemon essential oil on the chest.

A cup of sage tea made after the leaves are steeped in boiling water and then strained is another favorite remedy for soothing the throat. If you cannot find fresh sage in your local health food or herbal shop, buy it in tea bag form. If you want to use sage oil, remember that it is distilled directly from sage leaves and has a high level of toxicity. It is therefore advisable to dilute only a few drops in a glass of water when using it as a mouthwash.

A sore throat may also be caused by sleeping with your mouth open. If so, a bedroom humidifier will put moisture into the air as will steaming up the bathroom and inhaling the steam several times a day. Either hot-water steam or a cool mist will do the trick. If you have a respiratory problem or skin condition, ask your physician if a humidifier is right for you. A clogged nose may be another reason you are breathing through your mouth, causing a dry throat. If a clogged nose is the culprit, try using a decongestant nasal spray. While liquids will keep your throat moist, citrus juices are irritating and milky fluids produce mucus. Vitamin C and garlic tablets will combat the germs but if the pain and soreness persist, see a physician, as you could have strep throat, which requires medication.

AROMATHERAPY AND ESSENTIAL OILS

Due to the Taurean predisposition for sore throats and swollen glands, many essential oils can be used as mouthwashes, throat gargles, or soothing teas. Gargling with warm water combined with drops of geranium, lemon, eucalyptus, lavender, or myrrh—essential oils which correspond to Taurus and its ruling planet, Venus—works perfectly for sore throats, mouth ulcers, and inflamed, sore gums. Massage your throat, chest, and glands beneath the chin with sweet-smelling geranium, eucalyptus, and myrrh—the essential oil produced from the resin of the myrrh tree, indigenous to the Near and Middle East. In ancient Egypt, myrrh was noted for its rejuvenating qualities and, as a result, was used in the embalming process. According to Greek mythology, Myrrh, the daughter of the King of Cyprus, was transformed into a tree by Aphrodite/Venus, the Greek/Roman goddess of love and beauty. In her new form, Myrrh gave birth to the beautiful baby Adonis, whose obsessive love affair with the goddess proved fatal. To this day, Greek brides wear crowns made from the leaves of the myrrh tree to commemorate the love between Aphrodite and Adonis.

MINERAL SALT

Also known as sulfate of soda, sodium sulphate (nat. sulph.), the mineral salt recommended for Taurus, prevents water retention, regulates water supply, and eliminates excess water. A deficiency in this mineral salt may produce sweating, fatigue, and a tendency toward listlessness and depression. Foods rich in sodium sulphate include lettuce, onions, beets, cauliflower, spinach, cucumbers, celery, strawberries, and apples.

AYURVEDA

Just as Aries fits the profile of the Pitta personality, Taureans are almost exclusively Kapha types, whose greatest gifts include stability, serenity, dependability, patience, and contentment. When out of balance, or under stress, "they can be stubborn, dull, lethargic, gain weight easily, overeat, and store water and fat primarily in the thighs and buttocks."[3] In addition, digestion is slow and metabolism sluggish. Kapha personalities may feel depressed and cold because they frequently do not watch their diets or exercise enough.

To accelerate the metabolism and restore vitality, the Kapha body requires warmth and stimulation without the use of artificial stimulants like sugar and caffeine. Substitute cocoa or ginger tea for the usual shot of morning coffee, and add a bowl of oatmeal, buckwheat pancakes, corn muffins, or dry toast. Increase the consumption of bitter foods like romaine lettuce, endive, and tonic water, which promote digestion, as well as pungent, spicy foods and herbs such as cayenne, chili peppers, onions, garlic, radishes, horseradish, and ginger, which heat the body and produce an outflow of liquids, thereby decreasing water retention. Add astringent, high-fiber celery, asparagus, cauliflower, apples, broccoli, cabbage, beans, lentils, pears, apricots, carrots, lettuce, mushrooms, and potatoes to stimulate bowel activity, high-energy levels, and more concentration. A proper diet will help diminish procrastination, inertia, oversleeping, possessiveness, intolerance of cold and dampness, bloating, and weight gain.

Eliminate oily, salty, and sweet foods (see Appendix II), which Kapha types love, as well as mucus-forming foods such as wheat products (bread and pasta), dairy products (milk, butter, and cheese), and sugar until you lose weight and mucus is expelled from the sinuses and lungs. These foods can be added later but only in small quantities. Avoid fried foods and nightshade vegetables like tomatoes, zucchini, cucumbers, and sweet potatoes.

GEM AND COLOR THERAPY

If you were born between April 20 and April 30, your birthstone is the diamond. It is no wonder that diamonds, which are under the auspices of Venus, Taurus' ruling planet, represent love and marriage. If you were born between May 1 and May 20, your birthstone is the emerald. Other gems associated with Taurus are zircon (imitation diamond), jade, tourmaline, and turquoise—blue and green stones, the colors associated with Taurus. Lapis lazuli, a beautiful blue semiprecious stone, is a Venus stone and the material from which the cave of Inanna, the Sumerian love and fertility goddess, was constructed. Using a blue-tinted lamp or wearing gems which are shades of blue are said to open up the throat, which, in turns, allows you to communicate more freely, especially with the object of your affection. Diamonds and zircon will also affect this area of your life in a positive way.

Chapter 4

Gemini the Twins

Remember to Relax
and Take a Deep Breath

♊

Gemini the Twins (May 21–June 22)
Ruling Planet: Mercury
Element: Air
Modality: Mutable

Positive Gemini traits and concepts: versatile, winsome, engaging, humorous, charming, communicative, writing abilities, adaptable, amiable, youthful, intelligent, brilliant, rational, networking, logical, ingenious, brotherhood, freedom-loving, inquisitive, and cheerful disposition.

Negative Gemini traits and concepts: changeable, irritable, high-strung, restless, two-sided, inconsistent, dishonest, irresponsible, immature, excitable, unemotional, frivolous, superficial, and spreading themselves too thin.

Parts of the body ruled by Gemini include the shoulders, arms, hands, chest, and lungs. Its ruling planet, Mercury, governs the nervous and respiratory systems.

Ailments include asthma, bronchitis, collarbone problems, nervous disorders, panic attacks, pneumonia, respiratory problems, shoulder, arm, and hand dysfunction, pleurisy, and tuberculosis.

Professions which display Gemini's love of and talent for verbal and written communication, connecting with people, and/or retail include speechwriter, journalist, media specialist, public relations consultant, administrative assistant, translator, performer, comedian, circus artist, word processor, advertising executive, import/export, retail, trader, and instructor.

GEMINI THE TWINS:
CHARMING AND SOCIABLE YET
QUIXOTIC AND ALOOF

Gemini the Twins, a mutable air sign, is wonderfully witty, intelligent, and sociable, yet diffusive and easily bored. Versatile, charismatic, and natural dilettantes, Geminis usually strike up a conversation with almost anyone they meet. An information junkie, you can always hold your own and even give the impression that you are thoroughly familiar with and knowledgeable about any subject under discussion.

Named for the Greco/Roman messenger of the gods, Mercury provides Gemini, the sign it rules, with dexterity, quick-wittedness, speed, and an inclination to chatter away. Like its symbol, the Twins, Geminis are unpredictable and capable of contradicting themselves in the very same breath. You are extremely high-strung, cannot be pinned down for very long, and often have so many ideas running through your brain at once that thoughts often run away from you. While it may appear that you plot your actions and rehearse clever repartees, quite the contrary is true. You are, in fact, completely inspirational and your originality and inventiveness are purely spontaneous.

Geminis may be charming and have a way with words but are less than honest with their emotions. When it comes to speaking directly from the heart, you can suddenly become silent as a church mouse. Since pent-up feelings only add undue stress to an already tense and high-strung nature, one-on-one counseling, or talk therapy, is highly recommended for opening up and verbalizing your thoughts. Unlocking doors in an atmosphere of trust and relaxation is the first step toward openness and honesty. The key, however, is first to be honest with yourself; opening up to others will naturally follow.

Erudite and brilliant, the Gemini personality is also superficial and frequently undependable in an emergency. Yet you have an uncanny ability to adjust to any situation which calls for an instantaneous decision or a particular behavior pattern. On a positive note, if circumstances or situations become unpleasant, you won't think twice about making a switch or relieving boredom by taking on another project alongside a first. This does not mean that you can never hold a permanent job or carry on a long-term relationship. It simply means that to prevent mood swings and depression you must have several interests and outlets for your mental energy. It is important, however, to do each of them wholeheartedly—not halfway. Sometimes an inability to keep appointments or be on time is completely infuriating to your friends, yet you never lose your sense of humor, are the life of a party, and attract a wide circle of friends.

Because Geminis do not have long attention spans yet need to be busy at all times, they are normally involved with several activities simultaneously. Variety may be the spice of life, but

Geminis often spread themselves too thin to excel in any one endeavor. In fact, if you know someone who can iron, talk on the phone, and feed the kids all at once, chances are he or she is a Mercury-ruled Gemini—a jack of all trades and, all too often, master of none.

PHYSIOGNOMY AND BODY TYPE

Easily recognizable by defined eyebrows, wandering eyes, pointed nose and chin, and an angular face, Geminis are, more often than not, of average height and are quite thin. Always on the go, you normally appear agitated and restless; it is little wonder that Geminis stand out in a crowd.

Your ability to burn calories quickly and effortlessly allows you never to worry about putting on weight. With no excess fat, a complexion which seems to stay wrinkle-free, and a naturally lithe figure, Geminis remain young in body and spirit, no matter how many years have passed since high school graduation. If you don't want to get depressed, avoid your Gemini classmates at all those reunions.

TIPS FOR HEALTHY EATING

Despite these natural gifts, Geminis do not take care of themselves very well and rarely find the time to prepare nutritious meals or exercise regularly. Given the fact that they never have enough time to cram everything into frenetic schedules, it is no wonder their eating habits are equally erratic and meals almost always unbalanced. It wouldn't be surprising if fast food was actually invented by a Gemini who had no time for a proper lunch break.

If, however, you must eat and run, some fast foods are better than others. Rather than grab fried chicken, burgers, and fries, opt for a salad bar which offers a choice of raw vegetables, fruits, fish, and broiled chicken. Avoid anything fried or covered in gravy or, for that matter, any other unrecognizable liquid. It is best to use a salad dressing without mayonnaise such as oil and vinegar or a light vinaigrette.

Although a speedy metabolism and "constantly on the move" lifestyle prevents you from gaining unwanted pounds, loading your body with unnecessary fat and cholesterol could raise blood pressure and put undo stress on vital organs. Excess salt should be eliminated from your diet by utilizing a variety of salt substitutes or flavorful herbs such as rosemary, basil, dill, and thyme. While it is probably too much to expect that you will eat three square meals a day, five or six small meals spread throughout the day may provide you with the variety you crave.

As a Gemini, your greatest dilemma is learning how to strengthen, and not exacerbate, a high-strung, delicate nervous system. Because of a natural proclivity for parties and other social events where caffeine and nicotine thrive, Geminis find it difficult avoiding these and other stimulants, the use of which is associated with the ability to burn the midnight oil. Haven't we all seen old movies where the newspaper reporter or writer (Gemini professions) is seated behind a typewriter (now a computer) with a cup of coffee on the desk and a cigarette dangling from the mouth? While this image may have been romantic, what it represents is completely and utterly detrimental to long-term physical health and emotional well-being. Caffeine may be a stimulant which reduces fatigue in the short-term, but it nevertheless awakens the central nervous system, speeds up the heart and respiratory rates, and increases urine output. It brings on adverse heartbeat rhythm changes, which in turn results in increased nervousness, headaches, restlessness, irritability, depression, and insomnia—malfunctions to which Geminis are already predisposed.

CONQUERING INSOMNIA

If you cannot fall asleep easily or if you cannot stay asleep throughout the night, your problem may be insomnia. Although most people have periods when they toss and turn, Geminis are natural insomniacs whose minds work overtime even when they sleep. To counteract that tendency, you may try setting your body's clock by going to bed and waking up at the same hour every day. It is a good idea to avoid stimulants altogether, such as coffee, cola, chocolate (which all contain caffeine), and cigarettes, which will overstimulate the nervous system. Remember that if you do not get a proper night's sleep, you will awake more tired than you were at bedtime and your productivity will ultimately suffer. Rather than snacking late at night, drink a warm glass of milk and take a hot bath to induce sleep. Visualization exercises, deep breathing, yoga, soft music, and even sexual contact may help you to relax and have a good night's sleep.

When you do eliminate caffeine from your diet, remember that it is classified as a drug, and if you suddenly stop or limit your intake, you will probably experience minor withdrawal symptoms such as listlessness and "caffeine headaches." Rather than go completely cold turkey by avoiding not only coffee but cocoa, tea, soft drinks, and chocolate, try cutting back in increments. Have one cup of coffee in the morning and then switch to decaffeinated coffee, herbal teas, or caffeine-free soft drinks. They will not provide the same buzz but can be acceptable substitutes. I highly recommend Korean ginseng tea, a wonderful herbal stimulant that aids blood circulation and strengthens the nervous system without the aftereffects of tiredness and irritability once the caffeine wears off.

RESPIRATORY AILMENTS

Due to Gemini's rulership of the lungs and respiratory system, there may be a tendency toward bronchitis, chest colds, asthma, and, at the extreme, pneumonia and emphysema. Although fresh air and physical exercise are essential for anyone with bronchial problems, Geminis are more comfortable in the world of ideas rather than the physical universe. But they must learn that exercise and fresh air are essential to preventing and in some cases alleviating the effects of asthma and other breathing problems. Most Geminis will come to this realization if physical problems impede either their freedom or ability to be productive. If they persist in exerting themselves mentally while remaining physically inactive, Geminis may wind up with eyestrain, headaches, and even migraines.

LIVING WITH ASTHMA

Asthma is a chronic condition which arises when bronchial airways contract, causing tightness in the chest and shortness of breath, followed by coughing and wheezing. Asthma attacks resulting in the inability to control breathing are often triggered by allergic reactions to pollutants in the environment such as trees, weeds, grass, pollens, animal dander, dust mites, and mold. Additionally, episodes can be brought on by heavy exercise, viruses, and any form of stress. If you are asthmatic, give up smoking and avoid places where others smoke. If it is not an absolute necessity, do not venture outdoors in extremely windy, cold weather; if you do, use a scarf to cover your mouth. Moving to a warm, dry state such as Arizona was once advocated, and asthmatics moved there by the dozen. However, changes in the environment and the state's atmospheric conditions have caused an increase of dust in the air, and relocating there is no longer an appealing alternative for asthmatics.

Milk, eggs, nuts, and seafood are also thought to cause allergic reactions leading to asthma attacks. Other triggers are food additives such as metabisulfite and monosodium glutamate, more commonly known as MSG. It is a good idea to inquire before going to a restaurant if either of these are used and, if so, request that they be omitted from your meal.

For quick relief, most asthmatics use inhalers. It is advised that, rather than purchase them indiscriminately over the counter, asthma sufferers have inhalers prescribed by a physician, who can instruct them as to proper usage. Vitamin B_6, which calms the nervous system, may also be effective, but its intake must be approved and supervised by a doctor. If you are diagnosed as being asthmatic, familiarize yourself with the warning signs so you can intercept the onset before it becomes full blown.

If your attacks persist, seek medical attention immediately. Also, rid your home of all the above-mentioned pollutants, and repaint your house. If breathing symptoms (including cough, shortness of breath, wheezing, and sputum production) interfere with activities of daily living or ability to sleep, or if they persist for a long time, see a physician, since you may need medication either temporarily or permanently. If medication is prescribed, this does not preclude all the above-mentioned preventative suggestions, which should be used in conjunction with any prescription drugs.

If you are an asthma sufferer, the good news is that the condition is completely controllable so long as you take all preventative steps and properly prescribed medication.

DEEP-BREATHING EXERCISES

The inability to control fear, panic attacks, or an asthmatic episode may lead to hyperventilation, a condition marked by deep, rapid-fire breaths with no rest in between. This causes too much carbon dioxide to be exhaled, which may result in buzzing in the ears, dizziness, tingling of extremities, or even fainting. If you are prone to hyperventilating in response to tension, eliminate stimulants such as nicotine and caffeinated products such as coffee, tea, colas, and chocolate. The moment you recognize the signs that hyperventilation is eminent, namely heart palpitations and quick breaths, breathe into a paper bag so that lost carbon dioxide can be replaced.

The best method for relieving shortness of breath or hyperventilation brought about by stress, anxiety, asthma, or other respiratory conditions is the practice of Pranayama, the yogic science of breath control (see Chapter 2). With deep breaths, Pranayama opens the nasal passages and cleanses the lungs, thereby alleviating both physical and mental anxiety. Master this technique by attending yoga classes. Even though they may be initially resistant to learning a discipline which stills, rather than stimulates, the mind and body, restless Geminis will benefit greatly from the classes. If you do not have the motivation or the spare time to attend classes, allot ten minutes as soon as you awake and/or before you go to sleep for deep, steady breathing.

Deep, diaphragmatic breathing is another helpful method of relaxation. Whenever you are anxious or begin to hyperventilate, try the following exercise, which teaches you to breathe deeply from the diaphragm. (This is more or less how singers are taught to control their breathing.)

Step 1. Stand up straight with feet a few inches apart and arms hanging loosely at your sides. Head, neck, and body are somewhat relaxed. Shake your hands out to relieve any excess tension.

Step 2. Place your hands on your lower abdomen with your four fingers pointing toward your navel. This way you can feel your diaphragm drawing deep breaths.

Step 3. As you slowly inhale through your mouth, you are expanding your diaphragm and filling your lower lungs with air. At the same time you are doing this, raise your arms at your sides slowly, in a wide arc, until they are straight overhead with your palms together and your chest expanded.

Step 4. Hold your breath for as long as it feels comfortable.

Step 5. As you exhale slowly through your nose, turn your palms outward, lower your arms at your sides, and feel your chest and abdomen contracting.

Step 6. Repeat this process five times.

If you are not certain how your diaphragm should feel as it expands and contracts, place your hands on your lower abdomen with four fingers pointing toward your navel the first time you do this exercise. As you inhale, push your diaphragm into the palms of your hands. When you are ready to exhale, pull your diaphragm away.

Because Geminis need mental stimulation and social settings, you tend to become depressed, restless, and even anxious when alone. In addition to controlling the breathing and relaxing the body, this exercise in particular, and yoga in general, can be used to still the mind and alleviate anxiety.

The Importance of Good Posture

If most of your work is done sitting at a desk, it is imperative that you sit in a comfortable chair, since slouching may leave you with hunched shoulders and chronic back pain. Bad posture is not only unsightly (remember your mother telling you to stand up straight), it can lead to constant discomfort and disrupt healthy breathing patterns. When the body reaches a certain point in slouching, it "becomes frozen in bad positioning because the muscles have become unbalanced. Profound physiological changes have occurred, so you can't realign your own joints well enough to correct alignment without outside help. Once postural dysfunction has reached this stage, it is hard to reverse. You see this with people whose habitual posture is out of whack: They hold one shoulder higher than the other, or their back is swayed, or they can't hold themselves erect for very long without intense effort."[4]

Back and shoulder pain can be relieved by investing in an extremely comfortable chair that forces you to hold your back straight and lower your shoulders. Chiropractics, massage, and deep-tissue manipulation are methods for realigning your body. It is quite easy to maintain good posture for a few days to a week after you have a bodywork session. Many people, however, find they have to see a bodywork therapist on an ongoing basis to be reminded how it feels.

In addition, Geminis are adept with their hands and tend to type too fast or press too hard. Your natural attraction to computers means that you suddenly have to adjust your work habits in order to rest your eyes and your fingers. If you must spend long hours behind the computer screen, take five-minute breaks every half-hour. Stand up, let your arms fall to your sides, and shake your hands from the wrists. Otherwise you can wind up unable to work. In addition to getting a comfortable chair, make sure that you have a desk with a pull-out tray to accommodate the keyboard. If not, you may run the risk of developing tendinitis and carpal tunnel syndrome, which comes under the heading of repetitive strain injury (RSI).

REPETITIVE STRAIN INJURY

R epetitive strain injury is an umbrella term for several cumulative trauma disorders (including tendinitis and carpal tunnel syndrome) caused by overuse of the hand and arm. According to Dr. Emil Pascarelli of Columbia Presbyterian Medical Center, these repetitive hand movements which take place over and over again, each and every day, eventually strain and ultimately damage the muscles and tendons of the forearms, wrists, and fingers by causing microscopic tears as well as damaging the tendons, tendon sheaths, muscles, ligaments, joints, and nerves of the hand, arm, neck, and shoulder. Although RSI has been around for many years, mainly afflicting factory employees who use the same repetitive motion hour after hour (i.e., plucking chickens), the ailment has become an occupational hazard in newsrooms, law firms, and professional or home offices where computers are used regularly. Since Geminis are already prone to shoulder strain, it is a good idea to adhere to the following recommendations of Dr. Pascarelli.

1. Get a good chair in which you can sit comfortably with your knees at a 90-degree angle and your feet planted firmly on the floor. In order to accomplish this, the seat must be easily raised or lowered and your spine should be completely supported by the chair's back rest. Your spine should be correctly aligned, and your ears in line with your shoulders and hips.

The shoulders should hold the chest open, the arms support the hands above the keyboard, and absolutely nothing should be strained.

2. Get a keyboard you can reach with your hands straight ahead of you. Your arms should bend until they form a 90-degree angle at your elbows, while your middle fingers should line up with your wrists. If your desk does not allow you to maintain this position, then it is not the correct one to have. In lieu of buying a new desk, you can elevate your chair or insert the keyboard in a slide-out tray.[5]

3. Be certain that your computer monitor is level with your eyes so you don't have to strain your neck to look at it.

If you are uncertain how this works, stand or sit sideways in front of a full-length mirror to view your position. When you type, remember that your wrists, elbows, and forearms must never lean against the rim of the desk. Always pause at five-minute intervals to rest your wrists. These exercises will also help relieve, but will not completely prevent, the effects of arthritis, neuritis, and other degenerative ailments.

Vitamins and Minerals

Noted for the ability to strengthen and maintain a healthy nervous system, the vitamin B–complex group includes vitamin B_1 (thiamine), B_2 (riboflavin), B_3 (niacin), B_6 (pyridoxine), vitamin B_{12} (cyanocobalamin), vitamin B_{13} (orotic acid), pangamic acid, biotin, choline, folic acid, inositol, and PABA (para-aminobenzoic acid). Highly recommended to high-strung Geminis, this group of water-soluble substances cultivated from bacteria, yeasts, fungi, or molds provides the body with energy by converting carbohydrates into glucose and is vital to the metabolism of fats and proteins. Vitamin B is quite successful in treating irritability, depression, poor appetite, and insomnia. Most important, the B vitamins are necessary to promote normal functioning of the nervous system and may be the single most important factor for the maintenance of healthy nerves. Of this group, Vitamin B_6 is highly recommended for calming the nerves. (Never take vitamin B_6 on an empty stomach.) Foods rich in vitamin B include breads, rolls, whole-grain cereals, liver meats, soybean products, Swiss cheese, cottage cheese, and potatoes. Brewer's yeast, which is the richest natural source of the B-complex group, can be taken in pill or powder form. Although the powder has a lingering aftertaste, its unsavory flavor can be successfully camouflaged if added to cereal or fruit-flavored yogurt. Sometimes Geminis are drawn to starches such as bread, pasta, and potatoes without realizing that in actuality they are searching for something to calm their sensitive nervous systems.

Mineral Salt

Of the twelve essential biochemical mineral salts present in the human body, potassium chloride (Kali. Mur.), the one associated with Gemini, strengthens the respiratory area, prevents coughs and colds, and purifies the blood by maintaining normal blood-clotting levels and lowering blood pressure. Foods rich in potassium chloride include sweet corn, oranges, bananas, grapefruit, peaches, pineapples, plums, apricots, pears, green beans, turnips, collard greens, brussels sprouts, cauliflower, kale, lettuce, watercress, asparagus, carrots, and celery.

HEALING HERBS

Herbs and plants that strengthen the lungs and are, therefore, associated with Gemini include chickweed, saffron, anise, eucalyptus, fennel, heather, lavender, horehound, and licorice. Some of these may be added as food seasonings while others can be ingested in the form of tea.

If these spices do not fall within your budget (i.e., saffron) or are too exotic for your taste (i.e., eucalyptus), try adding everyday spices such as garlic or horseradish to your recipes. And if you can muster up the courage, eat a fresh clove of garlic or a tablespoonful of horseradish on a daily basis. This ritual cleanses your lungs and helps to prevent colds, fevers, and flu. Garlic's antibacterial properties have been prized since antiquity and its powers have been exaggerated to include protection against evil spirits. I was astonished in my travels along the Yugoslavian coast some years ago by the garlic cloves that hung on the doorways of almost every home to ward off vampires, werewolves, and other evil spirits who were supposedly chased away by vile odors. This type of folk remedy was very common throughout Eastern Europe, where Transylvania (home of Count Dracula) is located. It is also customary in some Slavic cultures for garlic cloves to be placed into the mouths, ears, and nostrils of corpses to prevent evil from infiltrating the dead. And in ancient Greece, midwives strung garlic from cribs and in delivery rooms to protect newborn babies from witches.

Teas made from borage (blood purifier and nerve tonic), lavender, licorice (diuretic and laxative), chamomile, vervain, and especially valerian are excellent sedatives and just as effective, if not better, for insomniacs than hot milk or counting sheep. Steaming your face with chamomile or eucalyptus tea clears the respiratory tract of excess mucus and works wonders for Gemini complaints ranging from shortness of breath to asthma to bronchitis and is a generally effective remedy for fevers, colds, and flu. The procedure for steaming is as follows:

Step 1. Place chamomile or eucalyptus leaves or ten drops of its essential oil in a large pot of boiling water. Fresh leaves are preferable, but if they are not available, tea bags will suffice.

Step 2. Cover the pot and let the tea steep for about five minutes.

Step 3. Pour the liquid into a basin and set on a flat surface.

Step 4. Drape a towel around your head and the basin so that your entire face and neck are completely enveloped in the steam.

Step 5. Continue for as long as you can tolerate the heat. After a five-minute break, repeat the process.

AROMATHERAPY AND ESSENTIAL OILS

Herbal fragrances and oils are especially helpful in treating certain ailments and conditions associated with a particular sign. Eucalyptus oil, an ingredient contained in many cough syrups and lozenges, relieves chest congestion and asthma if rubbed on the chest. After anointing this area of the body, be sure to cover the chest with a hot, dry towel to keep the person warm. Five drops of the essential oil of lavender, chamomile, or eucalyptus can be added to the bath for additional relaxation.

It is most important for Geminis to surround themselves with warm, sweet fragrances which expand the lungs and calm the nerves. Lavender has an incredibly sweet essence and works wonders to relieve painful stress headaches. Other therapeutic scents which come in bouquet form and can be spread around the house include basil, orange, rose, geranium, and cloves.

AYURVEDA

As an air sign, intellectual, nervous Geminis usually fit the profile of a Vata, or windy dosha. Symptoms of a Vata imbalance include worry, loss of mental focus, short attention span, depression, insomnia, fatigue, inability to relax, mental and physical restlessness, loss of appetite, impulsiveness, dry or rough skin, high blood pressure, and muscle spasms. Hiccups, asthma, respiratory complaints, and tension headaches may also be present. Due to this stress on the nervous system, it is most important for Geminis to learn to live more moderately, get ample rest, and set aside time for themselves. Regular massages and meditating daily are excellent ways to relax the body, silence the mind, and conquer insomnia. Other suggestions include avoiding drafts, eating three well-balanced meals, drinking hot, herbal teas throughout the day, and taking a warm, leisurely bath in the evening to calm the nerves and induce sleep. Each meal should begin with fresh ginger to stimulate the appetite and aid digestion.

One of the most important elements of Ayurveda is incorporating a diet specific to your particular dosha, which in this case is Vata or wind. Because of their high-strung natures, Geminis have very sensitive digestive systems which are usually aggravated by bitter, pungent, or spicy food. This sensitivity makes it difficult to digest high-fiber foods, including fruits and raw vegetables. Stews, soups, and hot, well-cooked vegetables are more beneficial than eating salads. Foods that soothe rather than aggravate the digestion will also ease the nervous system and help to win the battle against insomnia. The diet should include warm milk, cream, soup, hot cereal, and fresh whole-grain bread. Be sure each day starts with a hot breakfast. Due to the warmth of oil, eating fried foods is acceptable as long as it is not taken to excess. Spices such as ginger, cinnamon, fennel, and cardamom (used in Indian cooking) will help digestion and stimulate the appetite.

GEM AND COLOR THERAPY

If you were born from May 21 to May 31, your gemstone is the emerald; if you were born between June 1 and June 22, your gemstone is the pearl. Other gems associated with Gemini are agate, beryl, opal, and tiger's eye. For these particular gemstones to provide optimum effects, they must touch your skin and be set in silver, the metal associated with Mercury, Gemini's ruling planet.

Colors associated with Gemini are yellow and orange, while green is assigned to your ruling planet, Mercury. Surrounding yourself with the color green, which rules the heart, will calm the nerves and make you more relaxed, compassionate, and generous. When you are tense, be certain to take walks in the countryside or, if you are a city dweller, strolls in the park. If possible, try to develop a green thumb by working in a garden or with houseplants. If you have access to a spa where light therapy is offered, bathe under a green light.

Chapter 5

Cancer the Crab

Just Don't Keep
Your Feelings Inside

CANCER THE CRAB (JUNE 23–JULY 22)
RULING PLANET: Moon
ELEMENT: Water
MODALITY: Cardinal

Positive Cancer traits and concepts are imaginative, intuitive, tenacious, good-hearted, maternal, impressionable, responsive, sensitive, emotional, resourceful, protective, compassionate, friendly, loyal, mediumistic, and gentle.

Negative Cancer traits and concepts are deceptive, unclear, oversensitive, touchy, overprotective, clinging, controlling, defensive, self-indulgent, overly emotional, living in the past, overbearing, and holding grudges.

Parts of the body ruled by Cancer include the chest, breasts, stomach, digestive system, and the alimentary canal. Your ruling planet, the Moon, governs the mucous membranes and mammary glands.

Ailments include stomachache, gastritis, heartburn, indigestion, food allergies, hiatal hernia, and lactose intolerance.

Professions which bring out the Cancerian's imagination, culinary abilities, love of homes and collectibles, and/or ability to help and care for people include musician, painter, computer programmer, caregiver, doctor, nurse, social worker, psychologist, physical therapist, nutritionist, chef, antique dealer, shopkeeper, swimmer, real estate agent, and marine biologist.

CANCER THE CRAB:
TOUGH ON THE OUTSIDE BUT
SOFT UNDERNEATH

Cancer the Crab is a cardinal water sign whose emotional fulfillment is derived from being part of a loving, cohesive unit whether at home, among friends, or at the workplace. Idealistic, imaginative, and dutiful, Cancerians will do almost anything for a friend or loved one at a moment's notice. In return, they expect as much, if not more, than they give. Since few can ever live up to these expectations, Cancerians are often disappointed.

A devoted and protective caregiver, your maternal instincts are greatly appreciated, especially by those who, over the years, have come to rely on you exclusively. Since it's much easier for you to give than to ask for assistance, codependency (whereby your actions and need to take charge encourage and often facilitate your partner's dependence on you) is one way to mask your own needs and vulnerabilities. While this pattern of helping may have begun innocently, Cancerians can easily become overbearing and domineering over time. (See Chapter 8.)

The fourth sign of the zodiac, Cancer is moody, depressive, and withdrawn when the pressure builds and life becomes too hard to handle. Like the crab who retreats into its shell, you may appear hard and tough on the outside but, in actuality, you are sensitive, tender, and unabashedly sentimental underneath. Whether real or imagined, you often feel under attack and that you must defend yourself against the outside world. Rather than take an aggressive stance and act impulsively, you ponder your actions and proceed with caution until you are certain you are on the right track. At other times, you build up an impenetrable wall of emotional defenses and withdraw until you regain your confidence. While this stance makes you appear distant, reserved, and even cold, this protective device prevents you from getting hurt.

Like your ruling luminary, the Moon, which goes through many phases, your moods vary from loving, responsive, and outgoing one moment to solitary and meditative the next. In your moments of reflection you are unnecessarily hard on yourself. Rather than move beyond past mistakes with an eye toward the future, you frequently choose to dwell on the past.

Due to your gentle nature, you are frequently plagued by constant insecurities, worries, and pessimism. While you feel things very deeply, you usually keep your true emotions hidden inside. On the one hand, your fragility prevents you from expressing any negativity such as hostility or anger. At the same time, your insecurities can prevent you from reaching out for love or friendship—rejection would be utterly devastating.

PHYSIOGNOMY AND BODY TYPE

Like the Moon in its moment of fullness, you have large, saucer-shaped eyes, a pug nose, full, thick lips, and a circular face. Due to the roundness of your face and your accentuated upper torso, you usually appear heavier than you actually are. Your legs, which may be thin and shapely, go unnoticed due to your full-bodied figure.

Some researchers believe that by classifying people into apple and pear shapes, potential illness is easier to pin down. If this is true, Moon children (as Cancerians are commonly called) like yourself tend to be top-heavy and therefore usually fall into the former category. Cancerian women usually have large breasts, while men born under this sign may have overdeveloped chests. Whenever there is weight gain, the extra poundage usually goes directly to the stomach. If you do not pay attention to this early in life, you will surely complain of midriff bulge or a large paunch long before middle age.

What sets you apart is a sympathetic look which reflects your kind-hearted and generous nature. Because of an imagination that works overtime, you tend to become lost in daydreams—even when others are speaking to you. Often misconstrued as nonresponsive, you are, in reality, cautious, shy, and communicate more with looks than with words.

UNDERSTANDING DIGESTIVE DISEASES

Consisting of the esophagus, stomach, small intestine, large intestine (colon), and anus, the digestive system, or gastrointestinal (GI) tract, converts food into the nutrients necessary for life. The process of digestion begins with chewing and swallowing food and ends when it has been thoroughly broken down, assimilated, and eliminated. Peristalsis describes the muscular contractions which move the food through the esophagus, stomach, and intestines. If the stomach is not relaxed due to physical and/or emotional stress, the food may be regurgitated, or sit in the stomach creating nausea, heartburn, or gastritis.

Digestive diseases run the gamut from the occasional upset stomach to disorders of the gastrointestinal tract, the liver, the gallbladder, and the pancreas. This also includes malignancies and chronic conditions like colitis, ileitis, and Crohn's disease.*

When the breakdown of the immune system due to virus or bacteria is combined with emotional distress, one or more parts of the digestive tract become upset, resulting in indigestion, stomach problems, and gas pains. If your eating habits are not altered, these complaints can escalate into more serious, and often chronic, gastrointestinal illnesses. The most common ailment in this category is gastroenteritis, an inflammation of the mucous membranes which line the stomach and intestines, resulting in a range of symptoms from nausea to vomiting, and from intense gas pains to diarrhea. While gastroenteritis can result from a diet containing too much roughage or other foods difficult to digest, it can also be caused by bacterial, viral, and parasitic infections found in raw or undercooked food.

Eating properly will not only eliminate gastroenteritis but prevent its recurrence. If you eat a great deal of dairy products, be certain that you pay strict attention to the expiration date on the label, which indicates the last day the store is permitted to sell the product. Meat should always be thoroughly cooked and

---

* Since Cancer rules the upper digestive tract, esophagus, and stomach, Virgo rules the small intestines and process of assimilation, and Scorpio rules the colon and process of elimination, these diseases overlap these three signs. For the most part, however, Cancerians are more prone to stomach upsets, Virgos to ailments affecting the small intestines, and Scorpios to conditions of the colon.

the intake of roughage or oily, fried, and spicy foods kept to a minimum. Replace carbonated beverages and coffee with soothing peppermint and/or spearmint tea. Mint tea will settle your stomach and, if taken in the evening, will help put you to sleep. If you become dehydrated after a bout with gastritis, it is most important to immediately replace lost fluid and electrolytes (including sodium, potassium, and glucose) by drinking water or fruit juice. If your pain persists and/or there is blood in your stool, consult your physician immediately as the problem can be more serious.

HEARTBURN

Heartburn is a burning sensation in the chest (near the heart) resulting from acidic juices traveling from the stomach up the esophagus. Also known as acid reflux, heartburn is usually caused by eating too much food too quickly under stressful conditions. If heartburn acts up even before meals, it may be a sign of a peptic ulcer, and a professional should be consulted.

To prevent heartburn, eliminate caffeine, chocolate, carbonated beverages, hot peppers, and fatty meat from your diet. Ginger, tonic water, endive, and romaine lettuce calm stomach upsets and stimulate the production of digestive juices. Gentian root tea can be prepared about a half-hour before mealtime by simmering a teaspoon of the chopped, dried root in a cup of water for twenty minutes. Stress reduction techniques which aid the digestive system and relax the stomach include biofeedback, yoga, acupuncture, and tai chi. (See Appendix II.) Acupuncture and acupressure may alleviate chronic gas pains and indigestion by clearing blocked energy channels and guiding the chi (life's energy) toward the digestive system, restoring the balance to a tense system.

Other gastrointestinal complaints include hiatal hernia and gastroesophageal reflux disease (GERD), which may or may not precipitate heartburn. The most frequent cause of hiatal hernia is increased pressure in the abdominal cavity produced by coughing, vomiting, straining, or sudden physical exertion that causes the stomach to "turn back" certain foods, which then flow upward into the esophagus. Other than antacids, taking two tablespoons of Coke syrup (which does not contain the added irritating carbonation) can settle your stomach; the syrup is available at most pharmacies. Chocolate, alcohol, carbonated beverages, high-fat foods (especially fried), and nicotine tend to exacerbate reflux and heartburn and should, therefore, be completely eliminated.

Although nonprescription antacids provide temporary relief of heartburn, their long-term usage can result in side effects such as diarrhea, altered calcium metabolism, and magnesium retention. (Magnesium retention can be serious for patients with kidney disease.) As with other nonprescription drugs, if prolonged use (longer than three weeks) becomes necessary, consult your doctor.

If you have digestive sensitivities (as do many Cancerians), be advised that alcohol, aspirin, aspirin-containing medicines, and other medications (particularly those used for arthritis) can cause stomach bleeding, ulcers, or inflammation. If you are a cardiac patient and must take aspirin, your doctor will probably prescribe coated Ecotrim, which will not upset your stomach as it does not contain salicylate. Always remember to follow the directions on all over-the-counter medications.

LACTOSE INTOLERANCE

Since you are extraordinarily sensitive, it is recommended that you be tested for food allergies, especially if meals and/or light snacks bring on belching, gas, constipation, diarrhea, nausea, or stomach cramps. Digestive difficulties are often caused by lactose intolerance, a condition which occurs when the small intestine fails to produce enough lactase, the enzyme needed to digest lactose, the natural sugar contained in milk and milk products. As a result, the undigestible lactose remains in the stomach, causing nausea, cramps, bloating, gas, and/or diarrhea. Symptoms usually begin about thirty minutes to two hours after ingesting dairy products, depending on an individual's tolerance level. Although not everyone born under the sign of Cancer will be lactose intolerant, it is not a bad idea to limit the intake of milk and milk products if you experience discomfort after consuming them.

While there is no cure, lactose intolerance can be controlled by substituting powdered or nondairy creamers, which do not taste too bad once you become accustomed to them. Soy milk and soy cheese are high protein, nondairy substitutes that are readily available in health food stores and highly recommended to the lactose intolerant and to those who must lower their cholesterol. There are also enzyme supplements on the market which help digestion and break down lactose.

If tests show that you must limit or eliminate dairy products from your diet, it is necessary to replenish the missing calcium and vitamin D, which are both vital for prevention of bleeding gums, brittle bones, and dry, cracked skin. In addition to mineral tablets, calcium can be supplemented with watercress, lettuce, broccoli, kale, salmon, or sardines. Some brands of orange juice have added calcium. Vitamin D, which is normally obtained from milk products, is also found in eggs and liver. Since sunlight helps the body naturally absorb or synthesize vitamin D, you may just need to spend time outdoors rather than worry about food supplements. Vitamin D can always be obtained in a multiple vitamin and mineral tablet, which should be taken daily.

BUTTERFLIES IN THE STOMACH

Although it is caused by an actual physical deficiency, lactose intolerance and other digestive problems are further exacerbated when the stomach or digestive system responds to stress. When you experience emotional highs and lows, the stomach often reacts, causing what is commonly called "butterflies." While we have all used the term at one time or another, few people realize this flurry of movement is a very real phenomenon, triggered by the production of adrenaline.

When you feel fear, adrenaline is released into your system, signaling the blood in your body to be redirected from organs like the stomach to parts of the body like muscles, which would need extra blood in a flight-or-fight situation.

Since Cancerians tend to withhold their feelings, the key to controlling a nervous stomach lies both in the selection of a proper diet and the stabilization of emotional reactions. Remember to treat your stomach gently at all times. Do not indulge in strenuous physical activity until you have had an opportunity to digest your food, waiting at least an hour after each meal. Limit your intake of caffeine and carbonated beverages. Cut down on meat since it is difficult to digest. Although a high-fiber diet is recommended to thwart constipation and generally clean out the system, too much fiber can create gas. Watch your consumption of the following high-fiber foods: bran, carrots, broccoli, cauliflower, and leafy green vegetables like lettuce and cabbage. These fibrous vegetables are valuable sources of vitamins, minerals, and cellulose, but in large doses can irritate your digestion. Instead of eating them raw, they should be steamed or boiled so they are soft and digestible. Be careful not to overcook, however, or the vitamins and minerals will be boiled away. Tomato salads are easier to digest, and carrots or spinach added to mashed potatoes can be tasty.

STABILIZING EMOTIONS

In addition to eliminating the physical stress caused by digesting certain foods, it is important to lessen emotional anxiety, which can also upset the digestive mechanism. Rather than repress your feelings until they build up into fear, anger, or hostility, learn to express them without apprehension or guilt. Of course, this is easier said than done. One-on-one talk therapy once a week is a common method of delving into emotions. If your problem involves a partner, marriage counseling may be advisable. Additionally, your therapist (if you choose to go that route) is in the position to suggest a supervised support group where participants share feelings in a nonjudgmental, friendly, and supportive atmosphere. These groups are nonthreatening and you will not be prodded to divulge information unless you so desire. The goal is to learn to express yourself without fear, criticism, or self-recrimination.

HYDROTHERAPY

Literally meaning water therapy, hydrotherapy (from the Greek *hydro,* meaning "water") refers to any form of water work which alleviates complaints by soothing the nerves, easing muscle tension, and restoring general vitality. These include the application of ice, hot baths, saunas, steam baths, swimming, whirlpools, Jacuzzis, sitz baths, and even colonics (a special process by which water flushes waste from the colon). As a water sign, you already have a strong attraction to the seashore and water sports. You may not have realized that walking along the beach and sailing can be therapeutic, or that swimming laps exercises the muscles and eases stress by producing endorphins, which provide a feeling of well-being.

MINERAL SPRINGS

Many health spas and sanitoriums throughout the United States and Europe (especially Germany) were originally built in towns which had natural warm mineral springs. For centuries, Europeans have enjoyed the therapeutic benefits derived from sitting in naturally heated mineral springs even in midwinter. Franklin D. Roosevelt put Warm Springs, Georgia, on the map when it was revealed that he used the town's mineral springs to strengthen his polio-stricken legs. (If I hadn't experienced the magnificent feeling of naturally warm mineral springs in the mountains of New Mexico during the winter, I would not have believed their benefits myself.) In addition to hot springs, most health spas and healing resorts offer indoor whirlpools, swimming pools, Jacuzzis, saunas, and colonics, to which most people, especially Cancerians, overwhelmingly respond.

A hot bath with aromatherapy oils can calm nerves and chase away stomach butterflies. Steam baths and saunas are invigorating and induce sweating, which flushes out impurities. Relaxing the lower part of the body can be accomplished with a sitz bath, which calls for immersing the pelvis and lower abdomen in hot or cold water while the upper torso and feet stay dry. This is also good for cystitis and hemorrhoids.

The following simple exercise strengthens the immune system and relieves gastroenteritis pains.[6]

1. Lie on your back atop a sheet or blanket. Cover yourself from the neck to the waist with two hot, wet towels which have been wrung out.
2. Wrap the sheet or blanket tightly around the towels and remain in this position for five minutes.
3. After that time, lift the blanket or sheet and add a fresh, wrung-out hot towel, placing it over the other two towels.
4. Slip the two old towels out so that the new, hot one is in place, making sure you are covered at all times.
5. Place a cold towel which has been wrung out on top of the new, hot towel, then remove the hot towel so that the cold one is against the skin.
6. Rewrap yourself in the sheet or blanket. Add another blanket if you are cold. Remain in this position for about ten minutes.
7. Remove the now warm towel and turn facedown, repeating the process while on your stomach.

Digestive troubles, often temporary rather than chronic, can be caused by toxins and impurities contained in foods. In fact, diarrhea, vomiting, or the inability to eat due to heartburn, indigestion, and/or gastritis is often the body's way of saying that it needs cleansing.

Fasting for one or two days can cleanse the body by promoting detoxification and may be classified as a form of hydrotherapy. Drink only water, herbal teas, clear bouillon, and fruit juice which is fresh and unsweetened throughout the day. It is most important to drink at least six to eight glasses of water so that you are certain to flush out wastes and toxins. The more liquids you drink, the less hungry you are. Be certain that you do only light exercise and that you do not drink caffeinated or decaffeinated coffee, due to the acidic content. Fasting may also ward off flu or cold germs. If you can manage to fast for one day per week or every other week (as some people do religiously), your system will have an opportunity to recuperate and regain strength. Be certain to eat fruits, vegetables, and rice a few days prior to fasting and eat lightly for the first few days thereafter. It is beneficial to continue to drink six to eight glasses of water daily lest you reverse all the fast's positive effects. There are many spas which offer liquid fasts in a controlled, supportive environment, ranging from a day or two to longer stays for those with weight problems. If you are overweight, pregnant, on medication, or suffer from a chronic illness such as diabetes, ulcers, or colitis, do not fast unless your physician approves. Never fast for more than a day or two without your physician's consent.

PREMENSTRUAL SYNDROME

With your ruling luminary, the Moon, governing the breasts and mammary glands, Cancerian women and those with the Moon prominently placed in their horoscopes often suffer from fibrocystic disease—swollen or lumpy breasts which usually appear seven to ten days before the onset of menstruation. Fibrocystic disease is caused by rising levels of estrogen during the latter part of the menstrual cycle. If you are prone to this, eliminate high-fat foods and add high-fiber foods, which counteract the effects of estrogen. Avoid caffeinated food and beverages, which include tea, coffee, cola, chocolate, and cocoa, if you are prone to this uncomfortable condition.

Other common symptoms of premenstrual syndrome brought about by hormonal changes during the reproductive years are emotional distress, moodiness, and/or bloating. If you suffer from any or all of these conditions, you may benefit from the following premenstrual regime.

1. *Primrose oil*—Utilized for premenstrual syndrome and fibrocystic breasts, evening primrose oil, available in capsule form, is extracted from primrose seeds, which were once gathered by Native Americans for food. They are a rich source of GLA, a fatty acid which the body does not manufacture and yet is essential to good health.
2. Vitamin E—Take at least 400 to 800 mg per day for one week before you are due to menstruate.
3. Vitamin B_6—To ease the nervous system, you can take up to 200 mg during the week before onset of menstruation.
4. Magnesium—500 mg per day.

Herbal diuretics, like senna leaves and pennyroyal, which rid the body of excess water and ease premenstrual bloating, should be used sparingly. If steeped as tea, one cup per day is sufficient. Too many cups of herbal diuretics will cause cramps and place undue pressure on the kidneys and an already sensitive stomach. (See Chapter 8.)

HEALING HERBS

Whether in the form of after-dinner digestive aids, soothing tea, or a sprig of fresh leaves, mint is a wonderfully aromatic herb which grows wild in the Mediterranean region or can be planted in your garden. Its ability to settle the stomach and calm the nerves makes peppermint and spearmint primary ingredients in herbal tea mélanges advertised as having the ability to relax and tranquilize.

The word *mint* is derived from the Greek nymph Mintho, who, according to legend, was transformed into the fragrant plant by Persephone, who was envious of the attraction her husband, Hades, lord of the underworld, had for Mintho. Anyone who has ever smelled fresh mint can attest to the fact that its aromatic and refreshing odor alone can make you feel exhilarated.

Since you may be prone to indigestion, gas pains, and other digestive impairments, it is a good idea to keep fresh mint leaves in the kitchen cabinet at all times. Whenever your stomach begins acting up, steep the leaves in boiling water, strain, and a cup of hot, soothing tea is yours at a moment's notice. In addition to its therapeutic value, mint tea is refreshing, noncaffeinated, and tasty—and one of my favorite hot beverages. Whenever I have an upset stomach, or wish for a peaceful night's sleep, I turn to a pot of peppermint or spearmint tea for help.

Peppermint essential oil can be massaged onto the gums, teeth, and temples to relieve bleeding, toothache, and tension headaches. Inhaling the essential oil, adding it to a hot bath, or rubbing it on the affected areas may also alleviate (but not cure) pain brought about by neuralgia, arthritis, and rheumatism since it calms and strengthens the nerves and muscles. Peppermint ointments and oils are recommended to ease the burning sensation and pain caused by cuts, burns, and bruises. Rubbing peppermint oil onto the stomach will help ease digestive woes.

Healing herbs which assist digestion and counteract water retention include arrowroot, balm, bilberry, caraway, cloves, fenugreek, fennel, lovage, mustard, and pulsatilla. Angelica, in the form of roots and seeds, stimulates the digestive juices and relieves heartburn and stomach complaints. Arrowroot, a common wheat substitute available in powder form, is effective in calming the stomach and relieving nausea, especially when added to yogurt, cereal, puddings, or gravies. Used in herbal tea and known for their mild sedative properties, balm leaves soothe the stomach, ease digestion, and quiet the nerves. Chamomile is a wonder herb for tranquilizing the nerves, relieving congestion caused by mucus, and aiding digestion. (See Chapter 4.) Cloves in seed or oil form will take the edge off a long, hard day. Clove tea can relieve nausea and gas and purify the system. Fenugreek seeds and sprouts are also good in salads.

Utilized in Chinese herbal medicine, licorice root is one of the world's most widely used medications for the treatment of asthma, ulcers, and gastritis. It is available as a tea, in capsule form, and/or as a great aromatherapy oil. In southern Europe, drinking licorice water is believed to purify the blood.

Like anise and other mints, fennel is an after-dinner digestive aid which can prevent heartburn and indigestion. In India, fennel seeds are served at the end of a meal. If you have ever eaten in an Indian restaurant, you will recall that a dish of fennel seeds is either brought to the table at the conclusion of the meal or left out on the counter next to the cash register. Other than ingestion of the seeds, fennel essential oil can be massaged onto the stomach to relax the nerves and facilitate digestion. It can also be used to relieve hiccups, nausea, vomiting, and general stomach upsets. Other oils which aid indigestion, and settle stomachs when inhaled, placed in a bath, or rubbed onto the abdomen, include lavender (a popular all-around essential oil), peppermint, marjoram, jasmine, and verbena (better known as lemongrass).

Mineral Salt

Also known as fluoride of lime, calcium fluoride is the mineral salt associated with Cancer and is essential for tissue linings, the mucous membranes, and for the maintenance of bones, skin, and teeth. Without this salt, the bones will become brittle and the skin cracked and dry. Foods rich in this mineral salt are cabbage, kale, milk, cottage cheese, prunes, watercress, meat, egg yolks, rye flour, raisins, oranges, lemons, onions, leeks, and cheese.

AYURVEDA

Cancerians have a proclivity for water retention, which can lead to stomach bloating and, if the mucous membranes fill with water, lung congestion or asthma. Even if you are not lactose intolerant a mucus-free diet, which involves eliminating dairy products, is thought by some to eradicate excess fluids from the body. Although others maintain that dairy products have little to do with mucus, those who adhere to an Ayurvedic diet would completely disagree.

Like Taureans, stocky, lethargic, dreamy, and water-retaining Cancerians can be classified as Kapha types. Since your metabolism and digestive system may be sluggish, eliminate Kapha-aggravating foods such as fried, heavy (like red meat), and those high in sugar and fat. Unlike Taureans, however, Cancerians have extremely sensitive digestive systems and, as such, it is not recommended that they eat spicy foods or too much roughage.

Cancerians should strive to exercise regularly. Since they thrive near water, swimming, a highly recommended form of exercise which can be done year-round, is the perfect sport for burning excess calories while strengthening and relaxing the stomach muscles. It is important that six to eight glasses of water be consumed daily in addition to fresh fruit juices and herbal teas. It is advisable that fresh herbs for tea be on hand as well as a juicer for making fresh fruit and vegetable juice. (For Ayurvedic dietary and exercise tips for Kapha types, see Chapter 3.)

GEM AND COLOR THERAPY

The colors associated with Cancer are silver, white, sea blue, and green. If you were born between June 23 and June 30, your birthstone is the pearl. If you were born between July 1 and July 22, your birthstone is the ruby. Other gems associated with Cancer are moonstone, opal, and crystal. The metals are silver, aluminum, and selenite. Flowers are white lilies, poppies, and roses. Cancerians find the seashore relaxing and pleasurable, especially musicians and artists, who find the landscape inspirational. In fact, I know several Cancerian musicians who use the sound of crashing waves in their compositions, and painters whose favorite canvases are seaside landscapes or abstract paintings in pastel colors.

Chapter 6

Leo the Lion

Watch out for Your Generous and Overworked Heart

LEO THE LION (JULY 23–AUGUST 22)
RULING PLANET: Sun
ELEMENT: Fire
MODALITY: Fixed

Positive Leo traits and concepts are industrious, workaholic, flamboyant, dramatic, creative, magnanimous, proud, leadership, passionate, self-assured, innovative, original, expressive, loyal, exuberant, ambitious, dependable, and daring.

Negative Leo traits and concepts are domineering, self-centered, lavish, selfish, arrogant, conceited, bossy, controlling, cruel, rigid, obstinate, excessive, narrow-minded, hedonistic, brazen, and temperamental.

Parts of the body ruled by Leo include the heart, back, spinal cord, and spine. Your ruling planet, the Sun, governs general vitality, and the circulatory system.

Ailments include heart disease, hypertension (high blood pressure), atherosclerosis, edema (water retention), and chronic back pain.

Professions which appeal to the Leo sense of drama, independence, organizational skills, authority and/or magnanimity include performer, director, costume designer, lighting technician, producer, jeweler, executive, office manager, entrepreneur, host or hostess, educator, lecturer, proprietor, and civil servant.

LEO'S EXUBERANCE
GETS YOU WHERE YOU'RE GOING

A fixed fire sign, Leo is the most proud, dramatic, egocentric, and generous sign of the entire zodiac. There are two types of Leos—the extrovert and the introvert. The extrovert Leo is endowed with an air of confidence and an outgoing personality that lights up a room. She loves being the center of attention and gladly accepts the accolades that accompany her triumphs. The introvert Leo is a self-sufficient loner who speaks only when there is something worthwhile to say. What both Leo types share is creativity, resourcefulness, and a never-ending zeal for life.

Leos are ferocious about working independently and maintaining complete control over their lives. Unfortunately, they usually think they know what's best for others, who do not always appreciate the supervision. As a result, Leos are often perceived as bossy, even dictatorial, though they think of themselves as indefatigable and unwilling to accept defeat. Despite obstacles and impasses, Leos always manage to regroup, get back on track, and forge ahead.

Whether extrovert or introvert, you enjoy wearing the badge of magnanimity but could never be classified as altruistic. Unless you get credit, adulation, loyalty, or financial remuneration, it's unlikely you will give of yourself without getting anything in return. Subjective, childlike, and, at times, narcissistic, you are always motivated by the need to be noticed and ultimately loved.

In fact, you may have to weather several broken relationships before you realize that life is meaningless without passion and intimacy. Like your ruler, the Sun, your ultimate wish is to shine and, at the same time, be the center of someone's solar system.

Like the lion who is king of the jungle, you are a born leader and rarely a follower. A perfectionist at heart, you are drawn to any discipline which demands originality, quality, and high standards. Exceptionally creative, innovative, and a true visionary, your organizational skills and penchant for guiding others makes you an invaluable worker. On the other side of the coin, you find it difficult to delegate responsibility and become a team player.

As a fixed sign, you are inflexible and usually adverse to taking orders. If you must defer to authority, you'll find a way to put a personal stamp on what you do while remaining true to your ideals and faithful to your cause.

PHYSIOGNOMY AND BODY TYPE

Leos have very well-defined features, which contribute to an aristocratic and even defiant air. Projecting an image of certainty, you walk with a definite gait, and dress regally so you will be noticed whether walking down the street or standing in a crowd. Leos are usually recognizable by intense, deep-set eyes, hook nose, thick lips, and pronounced chin. It is, however, your hair which often sets you apart from the rest of the crowd. Wild and unruly, it may be thick, like a lion's mane, or thin, yet hard to manage and never in place. You may be either short or medium in height, and average or slightly overweight due to a penchant for rich foods and a dislike of physical exercise. Your strong constitution, resiliency, and aversion to being incapacitated enable you to heal quickly and fight infection—even common colds.

Classified as Type A personalities, Leos are hardworking, ambitious, responsible, often ruthless workaholics who thrive on stress. You are distrustful, resentful, and angry a great deal of the time, as though the weight of the world is on your shoulders. If you do not calm down and learn to take matters in stride, the body parts Leo rules are likely to feel the strain in the form of chronic back pain, poor circulation, hypertension, and/or heart disease.

BACK PROBLEMS

Backaches are caused by a variety of disturbances in the muscles, tendons, ligaments, bones, or underlying organs. These can range from temporary muscle sprain and slipped disk to chronic pain and curvature of the spine. Besides arthritis, osteoporosis, incorrect posture, physical exertion, and lifting heavy objects, back problems are quite often the result of tension and stress, which your stubborn, willful, and unyielding personality seems to encourage. Haven't you ever noticed how many people who suffer from back problems are also rigid, demanding, and have the need to be in complete control? Sound familiar? If your body retains a degree of inflexibility, the vertebrae will not stretch, causing enormous back problems and chronic pain. Executive-type Leos who sit for long periods of time may wake up one morning with a stiff neck, aching back, and, worse, a slipped, or herniated, disk. It is absolutely vital that you take breaks, stretch, and treat yourself to an extremely comfortable and ergonomic chair, which will help to elongate and stretch the spine even in a sitting position.

ALEXANDER TECHNIQUE

Preventing neck and back pain can be as simple as practicing good posture while sitting and standing. The Alexander Technique, which involves elongating your head, neck, back, arms, and legs is a great method whereby parts of the body that have been crunched up for years are stretched and lengthened. Once you master the technique and start to practice good posture, you may even discover that your body has attained its actual height, which is usually an inch taller than you think it is.

My Alexander teacher suggested that I visualize myself as a graceful swan, which helped me to angle my body to attain that image while sitting or standing. This particular technique is especially attractive to Leos (or Leo ascendants like myself), who have a natural affinity for role playing and pretending to be someone they are not.

At a height of five feet, it was very difficult to imagine myself tall and graceful, especially since I have always considered myself as somewhat clumsy. However, once I completed the initial visualization exercise and gazed into the mirror, I was amazed to discover that I actually had a longer neck and could hold it at a 90-degree angle to my shoulder. This technique has helped me enormously over the years since, more often than not, I sit at a desk for hours on end. Of course, it is easy to fall back on bad habits. So whenever I begin to slouch, I listen to a taped recording of an Alexander session, a reminder to realign myself, and once again I turn into a swan!

STRETCHING EXERCISES

For others, simple yoga and stretching exercises practiced daily may prevent, and ultimately eliminate, back problems by elongating your spine and providing general relaxation. These exercises, however, should be done as preventative measures before the onset of excruciating, constant pain. If you are already experiencing constant lower back pain, consult your doctor before you begin.

The following exercises supplied by my osteopath can be done daily. Remember to stretch only as far as you can and to stop immediately if you feel any pain. If you do these exercises over a period of weeks, you will gradually be able to extend your limbs farther and farther.

BACK BEND

1. Stand straight, placing your hands in the small of your back.
2. Bend backward at the waist as far as you can without straining, keeping your knees as straight as possible.
3. Slowly return to the upright position.
4. Repeat ten times.

PELVIC TILT

1. Stand with your back to a wall.
2. Bend your knees and keep your feet flat on the floor, shoulder length apart.
3. Keeping the rest of your body relaxed, tighten your abdominal muscles and tilt your pelvis so that the curve of the small of your back is flat against the wall.
4. Tighten your buttocks muscles.

5. Hold for ten seconds and then once again relax.
6. Repeat ten times.

KNEE RAISE

1. Lie flat on your back with knees bent at a 90-degree angle and feet flat on the floor.
2. Do a pelvic tilt by raising your knees slowly to your chest one at a time.
3. Hug your knees gently.
4. Lower your bent legs one at a time. Do not straighten your knees.
5. Repeat ten times.

PARTIAL PRESS UP

1. Lie facedown on a soft, firm surface with your arms at your side and head turned either to the left or right.
2. Keep your body still and stay completely relaxed.
3. Using the muscles in your back, not arms, raise your upper body enough to lean on your elbows. Stay resting on your elbows and let your lower back and your legs relax as much as you can.
4. Hold this position for thirty seconds at first, gradually working up to five minutes.
5. Repeat ten times.

YOGA POSITIONS

The Plow Pose, a popular yoga asana, or pose, is one segment of the more complex Sun salutation which yoga adepts perform at sunrise to greet the new day. Since the Sun is your ruling planet, this asana may be particularly appealing. Just like the Cobra Pose (see Chapter 8), the Plow is especially suited to elongating the spine and relaxing the body. Remember to stretch only as far as you can, inhaling and exhaling as you do each exercise. Practicing these yoga asanas on a regular basis will enable you to stretch a little more each week.

PLOW POSE (FIG 6.1)

The plow pose is vital for stretching the spine and strengthening and relaxing the back, neck, and shoulders.

1. Lie down on your back.
2. Bend from the pelvis and bring both legs down over the head.
3. Keep your legs stretched straight out through the heels so that they are at a right angle to the torso. Lengthen the spine. Remember to keep breathing.
4. Extend your arms and place them behind your head.
5. Allow your legs to go back only as far as you feel comfortable without collapsing the spine or chest. Be careful not to put too much strain on the neck. (If you feel pain, slowly release and come out of the pose.)
6. To finish, bring your legs down, exhale, bend your knees, and support the lower back with your hands. Straighten the spine slowly with the knees bent until you are lying flat.
7. Relax by remaining in this position with your eyes closed for at least five minutes. Continue to inhale and exhale.

These exercises and asanas may actually decrease your stress level, stretch your muscles, and prevent the onset of further back pain if done regularly. Additional relaxation tips include treating yourself to a massage several times a month. Since you crave at-

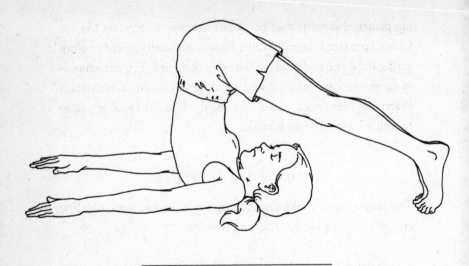

FIGURE 6.1 PLOW POSE

tention, you will love being pampered and comforted, while circulation is improved and tension alleviated. A theater-loving Leo such as yourself should also have no problem practicing guided imagery techniques as a way to relax and achieve serenity.

Other preventative measures for back pain include taking vitamin B to strengthen nerves, sleeping on a hard mattress, getting adequate exercise, and practicing good posture, like proper lifting by bending at the knees and not the waist. Most of all, avoid unnecessary physical and emotional stress. Acupuncture and massage help you to relax and to release tension so that energy may flow freely up and down the spine. Over-the-counter painkillers or anti-inflammatories help for a limited amount of time. Stop taking them immediately if you have stomach upsets, ulcers, or heartburn. As an alternative, white willow bark is a natural salicylate which just might do the trick.

If back pain persists, stop all medication and alternative therapy, including acupuncture, massage, and chiropractics, and see your physician immediately.

A herniated, or slipped, disk, to which Leos can be prone, is caused by a vertebra which has actually slipped, causing inflammation of the muscle on either the right or left side of the spine. I can vouch for the fact that a sudden slipped disk is no fun and, in fact, more excruciating than I ever could have imagined. One day I awoke and could not move a muscle. My husband had to gently pull me out of bed after I managed to roll over on my side in the fetal position—the only movement I was able to make. I followed my first impulse, which was to apply a heating pad to the afflicted area, and lie on my back the entire day. When I finally visited the doctor, I discovered that I had been on the wrong track. He prescribed anti-inflammatories plus ice packs several times a day. I was warned that, while strenuous exercise should be avoided, lying still would atrophy the muscles even further. He advised me to walk around and attempt my normal activities, but cautioned me to lie down the moment I felt pain until I was ready to once again get up and move around. I have since bought an ergonomic desk chair, which allows my back to naturally lengthen and elongate. I also do stretching exercises and Alexander Technique regularly while sitting and standing to keep my spine properly aligned.

PREVENTING HEART ATTACK AND STROKE

If, like many Leos, you tend to overwork without the proper rest, operate under a great deal of stress, are quick to anger, and tend to be overweight, you may be a perfect candidate for hypertension, one of the culprits which bring on a heart attack or stroke. More commonly known as high blood pressure, hypertension occurs when the heart is overworked as the blood moves through the body. Blood pressure is signified by two numbers— the diastolic pressure (the higher number on top), which measures arterial pressure when the heart contracts, and the systolic pressure (lower number on bottom), which measures pressure between heartbeats when the heart relaxes. The risk of heart attack increases if blood pressure rises above 140/90.

If you throw in obesity, nicotine use, a high-fat diet, and/or physical inactivity, a heart attack could be the ultimate result. Biofeedback (see Appendix II) can help to reduce your stress level and keep blood pressure down by heading off an emotional outburst or anxiety attack before it actually occurs. If you are able to recognize early symptoms such as sweating and heart palpitations, you may have time to utilize deep breathing and relaxation techniques, thereby nipping potential heart ailments in the bud. Since biofeedback requires a hookup to certain instruments which monitor physical reactions, I recommend that you attend classes or buy a machine for home use before attempting to recognize symptoms on your own.

Though some experts disagree on the correlation between sodium and hypertension, it is still advisable to keep salt intake to a minimum since it does cause water retention (edema), making circulation more difficult and increasing the likelihood of heart attack, stroke, and/or kidney failure. You may be unable to imagine life without automatically reaching for the salt shaker, but most people who have eliminated salt from their diets do not feel they have sustained a loss at all. Substituting spices and herbs such as black pepper, fresh garlic, thyme, sesame salt, and basil will soon make you forget you ever seasoned food with salt at all. You may also enjoy experimenting with a wide variety of exotic herbs and spices.

In addition to refraining from salt usage, it is advisable to limit ingestion of foods containing natural sodium such as cheese, soy sauce, margarine, nuts, smoked foods, and salty snacks. If you crave pretzels and chips, look for these products in salt-free or low-salt versions. Processed foods and delicatessen meat, which contain preservatives such as sodium nitrite, should be avoided. As a counterbalance, high potassium foods such as bananas, apples, oranges, potatoes, and fish are recommended as a means of maintaining low blood pressure and reducing the threat of hypertension.

LISTEN TO YOUR HEART

Heart disease is often hereditary and, if it does run in your family, do not aggravate your predisposition by consuming foods that contain high levels of cholesterol, which blocks the arteries leading to the heart, or putting undue pressure on the heart muscle through stress, obesity, and hypertension (high blood pressure). Even if you are not genetically prone, do not suffer from high blood pressure, or are not classified as a Type A personality, you may have other risk factors for cardiovascular disease. The good news is that these factors—smoking, high blood cholesterol, obesity, and physical inactivity—are easy to remedy as long as you are willing to make some lifestyle changes.

Because Leos love hosting and attending social functions, you probably eat large quantities of rich foods without paying much attention to cholesterol levels. Since, according to the American Heart Association, high cholesterol causes the majority of heart attacks, it is of utmost importance to understand the connection since you may be genetically or, at least, astrologically predisposed.

Atherosclerosis (hardening of the arteries), the most immediate cause of heart attacks, can result when excess cholesterol in the form of plaque begins to clog an artery, or arteries, leading to the heart. As the arterial wall narrows and is unable to pump blood into the heart, the ensuing sharp chest pain, called angina (short for angina pectoris), is a warning sign that trouble is brewing. If the artery should become completely closed off, or if a clot forms where the plaque is located, the blood supply cannot reach part of the heart muscle and a heart attack ensues. If an artery to the brain becomes blocked, the result is a stroke.

To prevent atherosclerosis and possible coronary disease, it is imperative to lower "bad" cholesterol and raise "good" cholesterol levels in the blood—both manufactured by the body. Derived from animal fat, bad cholesterol sticks to the arteries and is transported through the blood by low-density lipoproteins (LDL). Good cholesterol, carried by high-density lipoproteins (HDL), takes excess cholesterol from plaque-infested arteries to the liver, where it is passed from the body. Many experts believe that a high level of HDL, or good cholesterol, can counteract the effects of a high level of LDL, or bad cholesterol.

The following steps are recommended for reducing cholesterol levels in the blood:

- Restrict foods high in LDL or bad cholesterol such as red meat (especially liver, kidney, and other organ meat), shellfish (lobster, shrimp, scallops, etc.), dairy products (cheese, egg yolks, whole milk, butter, etc.), and saturated fats, including coconut oil, palm oil, palm kernel oil, butter, and cocoa butter.
- Substitute high-protein, low-cholesterol foods such as poultry (cut off visible fat), fish (other than shellfish), veal, egg whites, soybeans, and low-fat dairy and skim-milk products.
- Increase high-fiber foods, including fruits, vegetables, whole grain, and enriched breads and cereal. They will keep your weight down as well as raise the level of good cholesterol.

When eaten in large amounts, certain types of fiber, such as pectin and oat bran, may reduce LDL.

- Sardines, herring, tuna, and salmon oil are excellent sources of good cholesterol.
- Restrict your use of butter. Instead of saturated fats, substitute polyunsaturated (safflower, sesame, sunflower, corn, and soybean) and monounsaturated fats (olive oil, canola oil, peanut oil) since they lower the bad cholesterol and allow the good HDL to remain untouched.

Low-fat Cooking Tips

In addition to obtaining recipes from cookbooks which specialize in low-fat cooking, the following are some personal suggestions for lowering cholesterol.

- Mix skim milk, fresh fruit, a low-fat sweetener, and several ice cubes in a blender for a refreshing malted.
- Use low-fat cottage cheese, ricotta, skim-milk mozzarella, and other low-fat and nonfat cheeses whenever possible.
- Substitute low-fat or nonfat yogurt for mayonnaise in salad dressings. My favorite salad dressing, which I call creamy vinegar, consists of yogurt, vinegar, lemon, garlic, and black pepper. This dressing is basically Italian dressing with yogurt as a substitute for oil.
- Sauce made of fresh tomatoes, garlic, black pepper, thyme, and basil will help you forget rich cream sauces.
- Use egg whites instead of egg yolks.
- Instead of deep frying, lightly sauté in olive oil.
- Experiment with Chinese dishes which only require a bit of peanut oil, lemon, ginger, and garlic for seasoning. Lemongrass oil, which is commonly used in Chinese cooking, is also

thought to lower cholesterol levels. Go easy on the soy sauce since it is very high in sodium.

Some experts have suggested that blood cholesterol levels may be reduced by drinking one or two glasses of red wine or grape juice a week. Also recommended are high doses of vitamin-B complex, vitamin C, vitamin E, calcium, and zinc, which can all be obtained from foods high in these nutrients or in pill form. Lecithin, a nutrient found in soybeans, corn, cabbage, calf's liver,* cauliflower, eggs, garbanzo beans (chickpeas), green beans, lentils, rice, and split peas, helps breaks down cholesterol. Garlic is also said to reduce cholesterol as does tannin, an ingredient in certain teas, which, according to the *Prevention Book of Home Remedies,* prevents the conversion of simple fats into cholesterol. Both garlic and lecithin can be obtained in capsule form.

Lowering cholesterol levels is of utmost importance to every zodiacal sign but especially to Leos, who are astrologically pre-disposed to eating rich foods, being obese, inactivity, and expos-ing themselves to high stress—factors which lead to heart disease. If you have difficulty breathing or doing exercises which once came easily, get your cholesterol levels checked out at once.

While reducing cholesterol levels dramatically diminishes your risk of atherosclerosis, restricting your intake of fats helps to fight hypertension, diabetes, and obesity—all risk factors for heart disease. Fatty foods contain high amounts of calories and triglycerides—the form in which fat content occurs—even though they vary as to cholesterol levels. Margarine, for instance, may be low in cholesterol but contains as many calories as but-ter. This is true of saturated, polyunsaturated, and monounsatu-rated fats, which differ in cholesterol levels but are high in

---

* *Always remember that liver, an organ meat high in cholesterol, should be eaten sparingly.*

calories and triglycerides. Since extra poundage places additional pressure on the heart's ability to pump blood, and diabetes is aggravated by high triglycerides, consumption of both low- and high-cholesterol fatty foods should be curtailed.

It's a good idea to maintain the type of diet recommended by the American Heart Association, which consists of about two-thirds fruit, vegetables, cereals and whole grains, and one-third meat and dairy products. These recommendations should be followed by those who wish to maintain good health but are especially valuable for those who are predisposed to heart problems.

I know that you Leos reading this are going to rebel, as you believe that you can overcome anything by sheer force of your will. Unfortunately, the body is like an automobile; if you abuse it, the mechanism will simply quit. Although deviating from established habits does not come easily for any of the fixed signs, good health, vitality, and longevity should be your first priorities. Pride may, at first, prevent you from admitting that you are mortal, but vanity will ultimately motivate you to change your dietary habits and embark on an exercise regime. It is unlikely that you will allow anything to get the best of you—especially weight gain and illness.

The American Heart Association recommends thirty minutes of aerobic exercise, which expands and conditions the heart and lungs, at least three or four days a week to anyone who wants to stay in shape. Swimming, fast walking, running, jumping rope, calisthenics, and other brisk movements that increase the heart rate come under the category of aerobic exercise. In addition to strengthening the heart and lungs, brisk exercise burns calories, alleviates hunger, and lowers cholesterol. Other forms of movement, including leisurely walking, dancing, gardening, and performing household chores, will still burn calories and condition your body, but not to the same extent as aerobic exercise.

Once you decide to start exercising seriously, it is important that you recognize your physical capabilities and personal preferences. Since you like to be in complete control of your time, and have a tendency to keep long work hours, you may rebel against attending scheduled aerobics classes. Consider instead buying an exercise bicycle or treadmill for your home to use at your own convenience rather than adhering to class timetables. To get fresh air, running, walking, and bicycling are activities which can be done solo. Individual competitive sports such as racquetball and tennis probably interest you more than team sports like volleyball and basketball. (You Leos are not big "joiners.") Before embarking on an exercise program, it is important to see your physician, especially if you have already had a heart attack or back injury.

In India, *upayes* (Sanskrit for "remedial measures") are frequently recommended by astrologers to avert difficulties to which you may be prone. Aside from prayers, mantras (chants), diet, and gemstones to heal your afflictions, the simplest method is becoming charitable and opening your heart to others as good deeds are thought to literally expand the heart muscle. If you think about the happiness and tranquillity which is often derived from doing a good deed, helping someone less fortunate, or volunteering for a cause, this metaphysical lesson makes a good deal of sense.

AROMATHERAPY AND ESSENTIAL OILS

While each aromatherapy fragrance relieves stress, jasmine and juniper head the list. Used as bath oils, especially after a hard day's work, these scents will help you to relax. When massaged on the face and neck, they are known to vastly improve circulation. Jasmine oil is a wonderful perfume, a fabulous smelling incense, as well as a great-tasting tea. In any form, the unique, sweet smell of jasmine will quell stress, anxiety, and nervous tension. Eucalyptus, juniper, black pepper, lavender, or rosemary oil should be rubbed onto the back, neck, and shoulders to relieve pain and ease muscle tension.

HEALING HERBS

As we have already seen, certain herbs and spices are known to prevent, relieve, or even help cure certain ailments which are the domain of particular zodiacal signs. Circulation is aided by alfalfa, fenugreek, gentian, comfrey, thyme, and nettles, while herbs which prevent high blood pressure include rosemary, lavender, heather, and anise. Borage tea acts as a stimulant, antidepressant, and blood purifier. Dandelion, rich in vitamins A, B, and C, cleanses the bloodstream and functions as a diuretic. Rosemary, a popular, aromatic herb which reduces blood pressure and stimulates circulation, enlivens stews, soups, meat and chicken dishes, can be brewed as tea, and is a well-known emulsifying shampoo ingredient for dry hair. Vitamin E prevents high blood pressure and can be taken in tablet form or by eating wheat germ, sunflower seeds, salmon, peanut butter, broccoli, and spinach.

MINERAL SALT

Phosphate of magnesium (Mag. Phos.), the mineral salt associated with Leo, helps maintain normal blood pressure. It also promotes proper functioning of the lungs and nerve tissues. For Leos, who rely on their vitality, this mineral will restore lost vigor and strengthen muscles and blood circulation. Foods rich in magnesium are walnuts, onions, coconuts, plums, almonds, blueberries, cucumbers, barley, bran, peas, oatmeal, savoy cabbage, oranges, lemons, lettuce, figs, eggs, and asparagus.

AYURVEDA

As a fire sign, Leo, like Aries, fits the Pitta profile. Ambitious, industrious, and energetic, you are governed by the Sun, which, like Mars, ruler of Aries, is considered a fiery, Pitta planet. Although you are not as impulsive and physically daring as Aries personalities, you certainly thrive on industriousness, achievement, and productivity. Like Aries, you overwork to the point of exhaustion and generate a great deal of heat. Since Leos are ruled by the Sun, there is no question that a warm climate induces the greatest degree of comfort.

Since Pitta is considered a very "hot" dosha, opt for foods that are refreshing and will cool your body. Prepare salads rather than soups, and whenever possible eat raw vegetables. For breakfast, prepare cold cereal, cinnamon toast, and apple juice instead of hot cereal and orange juice. Avoid foods that are considered salty, sour, and spicy in favor of bitter, sweet, and astringent tastes. Stay away from pickles, yogurt, sour cream, vinegar, alcohol, coffee, or any other foods that are acidic and/or fermented. Refreshing beverages include peppermint and licorice tea. (For more information about Pitta diet, see Chapter 2.)

GEM AND COLOR THERAPY

If you were born between July 23 and July 31, your birthstone is the ruby, a precious red stone; if you were born between August 1 and August 22, the gemstone is the peridot. Gems associated with the Sun, Leo's ruling planet, include garnet, coral, rose quartz, and crystal quartz. These stones should always be set in gold, the metal associated with fire signs. For optimum effect these gems should touch the heart either as a pendant or worn against the skin beneath clothing. Rose quartz is said to bring love into one's life, and someone I know can personally attest to that.

Concerned that her daughters would never find true love, she began wearing three stones against her skin, one for each child. Before the year's end, two of them announced their engagements. Crystal quartz aids the blood circulation and restores vitality but can cause palpitations when worn too close to the heart. I for one cannot wear crystals for that very reason. Instead of providing energy, they make me feel as though I've had too many cups of coffee! If you are sensitive, rub the crystal in the palms of your hands a few times a day, or substitute a garnet, coral, or ruby.

The colors associated with Leo are yellow, the color of the Sun, and red, the color of blood. Stones associated with Leo all have a reddish hue. Placing yellow flowers like marigolds, daffodils, and sunflowers around your house will cheer you up if you are feeling down. With the Sun as Leo's ruling luminary, it is almost impossible for individuals born under this sign to be comfortable in a cool or rainy climate. As Sun worshipers, you must be sure to use strong sunscreen and stay out of the Sun for long periods or it will dry and chap the skin and cause rashes. Just basking in the heat of the Sun does wonders for a condition like SAD (Seasonal Affective Disorder), a state of depression which affects people in the winter when the Sun's rays are weak.

Chapter 7

Virgo the Virgin

Good-Natured, Critical, and a Bundle of Nerves

VIRGO THE VIRGIN (AUGUST 23–SEPTEMBER 20)
RULING PLANET: Mercury
ELEMENT: Earth
MODALITY: Mutable

Positive Virgo traits and concepts are kindhearted, gentle, intelligent, creative, research abilities, service-minded, efficient, loyal, detail-oriented, helpful, dependable, methodical, reserved, pragmatic, intellectual, animal-lover, and humble.

Negative Virgo traits and concepts are critical, self-conscious, cold, calculating, strict, fastidious, indecisive, manipulative, nervous, introverted, high-strung, overly analytical, absent-minded, and moralistic.

Parts of the body ruled by Virgo include the abdomen, digestive tract, solar plexus, spleen, and small intestine. Your ruling planet, Mercury, governs the nervous system.

Ailments include ulcers, intestinal disorders, digestive problems, diverticulitis, ruptured spleen, neuralgia and other nerve ailments, insomnia, and panic attacks.

Professions which illuminate the Virgoan love of detail, science, service, and organization include researcher, scientist, writer, editor, illustrator, chemist, physical therapist, social worker, medical caregiver, veterinarian, secretary, administrative assistant, accountant, bookkeeper, teacher, critic, and health food store owner.

VIRGO THE VIRGIN: METICULOUS AND CRITICAL YET GENTLE AND KIND

Symbolized by a young maiden holding a sheaf of harvested corn, Virgo, a mutable earth sign, is sensitive, gentle, meticulous, and service-oriented. In keeping with an altruistic and sincere desire to make the world a better place, Virgos are drawn to the helping professions. You might be an avid contributor and/or supporter of animal rights groups, like Greenpeace or other environmental organizations whose goals are to improve the quality of life. Your efficiency, organizational skills, and impeccable eye for detail are best served in a supportive rather than leadership role. To that end, corporate heads, entrepreneurs, and creative visionaries would be totally lost without the Virgos of the world, who ensure that projects are completed and carried out according to plan.

The desire to have others take credit while you stay in the background is, in part, due to modesty, self-consciousness, and, at times, self-deprecation. Fearful of being castigated for anything short of perfection, you can be extraordinarily judgmental, principled, and extremely critical of those (including yourself) who do not meet your high standards. While the demand for quality propels you to fulfill your goals, it often leads to dissatisfaction (with yourself and others), difficult relationships, and low self-esteem. In a quest for perfection, you tend to become obsessive about diet, hygiene, and exercise, and can compulsively overwork to the exclusion of relaxation and/or fun.

Utterly meticulous, critical, and painfully self-conscious, you are, at the same time, kindhearted, remarkably hospitable, and possess a strong sense of loyalty and responsibility. Like Gemini, you are ruled by communicative Mercury, named for the fleet-footed messenger of the gods, which provides you literary and verbal skills yet prevents you from being emotionally or physically demonstrative. Mercury's influence causes you to be discriminating, pragmatic, and highly analytical.

Unfortunately, you are your own harshest critic and, as such, judge yourself and others too severely. You find it difficult to express your feelings even to those who are close, and hesitate to initiate a project for fear that others will belittle your talents, opinions, and ideals. Quite often, you will commit to a project or an intimate relationship out of a sense of responsibility, obligation, or friendship rather than love and physical attraction. When duty calls, Virgo is the first to respond and the last to quit. Since you are not excessive like Taurus, Libra, or Pisces, you needn't feel guilty about letting your hair down once in a while. Enjoyable outlets may actually calm your nerves and strengthen your immune system—which high-strung Virgos with delicate systems desperately need.

VISUALIZATION EXERCISE

The following creative visualization exercise is a way to relax without any qualms or guilt about having a good time:

1. With eyes closed, find a comfortable position either sitting or lying down, and clear your mind of any thoughts.
2. Picture where you were and what you were doing the last time you truly enjoyed yourself without worrying what others thought. Perhaps you were dancing, partying, relaxing with friends, making love, or walking along the beach.
3. Once you have that image in your mind, re-create the sights, sounds, and odors which permeated at that time. If indoors, what were the colors of the room? If outdoors, what time of day was it and how was the weather? If you were having refreshments, try to remember the tastes. What topic was being discussed, if any? If possible, try to re-create and hear the conversation.
4. Once you have placed yourself back in time, try to recall the emotions and feelings you were experiencing. Were you fearful because you wanted to relax but could not? Or were you completely at ease, conversing or even laughing?
5. Try to recollect the sights, sounds, smells, and tastes of the moment and, most of all, how happy you were.
6. Keeping that image in mind, slowly open your eyes, retaining the feeling of well-being as you go on to your next activity.

Start each morning with this five-to-ten-minute visualization exercise. The memories of a happy time will help you to relax and enjoy yourself. By incorporating those feelings into your daily routine, your attitude toward life may actually begin to change.

Physiognomy and Body Type

Due to nervous energy and a speedy metabolism, Virgos are often lanky and lean. They have very fine, delicate features, kind yet restless eyes, small nose, thin lips, and are often fidgety. With so much always on your mind, you probably find it difficult, almost excruciating, to sit still. Although not usually robust, you are extremely health-conscious, and many hours may be allotted to physical exercise in aerobics classes or lifting weights.

Good eating habits, regular exercise, and plenty of fresh air are high on your list of priorities. With a sensitive digestive system and jittery disposition, it's likely that you chose to abstain from caffeine, nicotine, and alcohol long ago. Increase your intake of fresh fruits and vegetables, and try to find a way to decrease the emotional and physical stress which can irritate an already sensitive digestive system and intestinal tract. It is advisable to eat five to six small meals throughout the day rather than three large meals, which have the tendency to sit in the stomach. It is also a good idea to avoid eating gas-producing or spicy foods.

Many Virgos I know are either completely vegetarian* (no meat, poultry, and fish), or gave up red meat many years ago in favor of fish and/or chicken. Studies continually conclude that those on meatless diets have lower cholesterol and blood pressure than those who eat meat. Vegans, whose diet consists of no animal products whatsoever (including dairy products), must take vitamin B_{12} supplements.

If you are vegetarian, it is of utmost importance to make appropriate substitutions to ensure that the body has adequate pro-

---

Vegans are vegetarians who do not include dairy or any animal products in their diet, while lactovegetarians consume milk and milk products.

tein. Dairy products should only be eaten occasionally since there is a risk of raising cholesterol and fat if too many are consumed. In addition to milk, cheese, and eggs, protein requirements can be satisfied by eating:

- a variety of vegetables; legumes such as split peas, lentils, and chickpeas (garbanzos);
- whole grains such as brown rice, barley, and buckwheat;
- beans;
- soy products—all of which contain no fat or cholesterol.
- Nuts are good sources of protein, unsaturated fat, vitamins B and E, calcium, iron, potassium, magnesium, phosphorus, and copper. Although they contain unsaturated fats and, therefore, no cholesterol, nuts are high in calories.
- Pumpkin seeds, sesame seeds, and sunflower seeds are rich in protein and great for snacking. They also contain vitamins A, B, D, and E, phosphorus, calcium (especially sesame seeds), iron, fluorine, iodine, potassium, magnesium, zinc, and unsaturated fatty acids.

When switching to a vegetarian diet, it is imperative that your body is supplied with the 22 amino acids, or protein builders, eight of which are not produced by the body in sufficient amounts and, therefore, should be obtained from food. Although grains are protein substitutes, they must be combined with other grains, vegetables, or dairy products, to supply the amino acids necessary to create the "whole" protein found in fish, meat, poultry, and cheese. They need not be eaten together, however, since the body stores certain types of amino acids until their complements are obtained. The best combinations for deriving whole protein are as follows:

1. Legumes, beans, peas, and lentils with sesame and sunflower seeds.
2. Legumes, beans, peas, and lentils with grains. Under this category come beans and rice, lentils and rice, or beans on toast.
3. Whole grains with dairy. Under this category can be a cheese sandwich on whole grain bread, macaroni and cheese casserole, or rice and cheese casserole.

Tofu (soybean curd), tempeh (fermented soy), seitan (wheat gluten), and miso (fermented soy paste used in popular miso soup) are viable high-protein meat substitutes that can be used in dishes ranging from tofu lasagna to seitan "meatballs." Vegetarians who are lactose intolerant can opt for pizza topped with melted tofu, which provides the same creamy texture as cheese.

If you wish to pursue a vegetarian diet, an important tip is to vary your foods as much as possible. If you thought that soy and cheese were your only substitutes, you would not be providing yourself with enough nutritious choices and would get bored rather easily.

Seitan has the consistency of meat and, while its taste differs, will provide the feeling that you are chewing and digesting food that has more bulk than vegetables. Tofu is a perfect protein substitute since it is fat- and cholesterol-free, yet has an abundant supply of calcium, choline, potassium, and vitamins B, C, and E. Tofu can be added to salads, lightly sautéed to enhance the flavor, stir-fried with vegetables, and used as a meat substitute in spaghetti sauce, pizza, or lasagna. Combined with mayonnaise, chopped celery, and onion, tofu salad is a great tuna substitute.

A vegetarian diet automatically lowers your fat, cholesterol, and caloric intake since plants have little fat and/or cholesterol—a great boon to weight control. Don't substitute only cheese and eggs, which will raise your fat and cholesterol levels. Add substantial amounts of whole grains and vegetables to your diet. Some vegetarians eat fish, and those who follow macrobiotics, a specialized diet based on the Chinese philosophy of balancing yin and yang, vary their diet among whole grains, vegetables, and fish.

In addition to being easy on your digestive system, a vegetarian diet is high in fiber and beneficial for lowering the risk of heart disease, diverticulitis, ulcers, and other stomach disorders. Most people eat more protein than is actually necessary and do not realize that excess protein can exacerbate arthritis and kidney ailments.

Potassium is also very important for Virgos, as it activates production of digestive enzymes which stimulate the entire gastrointestinal tract and ease pressure on the intestines. In addition, potassium deficiencies, which are sometimes the result of excessive sodium intake or an insufficient amount of fruits and vegetables in the diet, can exacerbate the insomnia from which many Virgos suffer. Foods especially high in potassium include green leafy vegetables, strawberries, bananas, oranges, asparagus, cantaloupe, almonds, potatoes (especially the skin), sesame and sunflower seeds, and tuna.

Like Mercury-ruled Geminis, high-strung Virgos are often plagued by nervous tension, insomnia, and anxiety attacks. Strengthening the nervous system and increasing the threshold for stress can be attained through yoga, meditation, deep-breathing exercises, and creative-visualization techniques, which may take the edge off nervousness and irritability. By monitoring anxiety levels, biofeedback (see Appendix II) can warn that a full-blown anxiety attack is on its way. (See Chapter 4 for exercises for hyperventilation and recommendations for decreasing insomnia and nervous tension.)

Meditation, or clearing the mind of unwanted thoughts, is

the best way for Virgos to relax and calm the nerves. Although there are a variety of techniques which utilize mantras, sounds, and visual images to blot out thoughts, the simplest method involves focusing on the rhythm of your breath as follows:

1. Close your eyes and sit straight with your back against the wall. Direct all your attention inward, eradicating all thoughts. Try to keep your spine straight, releasing all the tension in your shoulders, neck, and face.
2. As you breathe, shift your energy by concentrating on the *hara* point—a few inches below the navel. (This is the point from which all physical energy emanates.)
3. Continue to concentrate on your breathing, allowing it to find its own rhythm.
4. After a few breaths, slowly exhale and visualize that your breath is flowing up your torso from your hara, through the shoulders, down the arms, and out the fingertips.

After doing this exercise for five to ten minutes, you should be relaxed and your mind should be free of troubling thoughts. You may already be experienced in other meditation techniques, so continue to practice what you find comfortable.

Your erratic temperament, mood swings, and high expectations accompanied by constant worrying, analyzing, and internalizing, make you a prime candidate for either temporary or chronic depression. Initial signals that depression may be near include lack of interest in sex, change in eating habits (i.e., loss of appetite or binge eating), fatigue, sadness, insomnia, and irritability.

Although you may not suffer from clinical depression, you have probably been plagued at one time or other by a tendency to worry, fret, and be generally pessimistic about the future. If you ask a Virgo to describe a glass which is filled halfway with water, the answer will invariably be that the glass is half empty, the mark of a pessimist, rather than half full, indicative of an optimist. Although artificial stimulants like caffeine can temporarily perk you up, their long-term effects include depletion of energy, accelerated mental activity, diminished concentration, and an even more vulnerable nervous system. In addition to B-complex vitamins and brewer's yeast (see Chapter 4), the following herbs are natural stimulants which strengthen the nervous system, thereby increasing powers of concentration and stamina. They also aid in the production of serotonin, a mood regulatory chemical in the brain which brings about a feeling of well-being and helps to control and relieve anxiety and depression.

GINSENG AND OTHER HERBS

Ginseng, a plant grown in Siberia, China, and Korea (that grown in Korea is considered the most potent), is a blood purifier and natural stimulant available as a capsule, in the form of tea, or as a tonic. The root has been utilized in Chinese medicine since at least the first century A.D. to restore vitality and as an all-round healer for almost every physical condition. Ginseng strengthens the heart and nervous system so that the body's response to stress is manageable, and anxiety is controlled before it escalates into a full-blown panic attack. Ginseng is said to enhance good health to such an extent that some people believe it inhibits impotence and promotes general longevity. The benefits lie in its ability to stimulate sans the nervousness which accompanies caffeine. Additionally, this herb improves the appetite, has a positive effect on digestion, and relieves stomach ailments.

Ginseng builds up vitality and resistance to disease by stimulating the endocrine glands, which control physiological processes such as the metabolism of minerals and vitamins. High blood-sugar levels are lowered by ginseng, which also effectively treats hypertension by normalizing the level of arterial pressure. In addition to its healing properties, ginseng contains vitamins, minerals, and enzymes. This herb is also used to treat colds, coughs, rheumatism, neuralgia, gout, diabetes, anemia, insomnia, stress, and headache.

The following herbs are equally potent for relieving both insomnia and depression:

Valerian—A popular herb, valerian comes from the same root as Valium (diazepam), a muscle relaxer once readily prescribed by physicians to quell anxiety and bring on sleep. Since it lacks Valium's addictive properties, valerian is much safer and just as effective when ingested regularly. It is readily available in capsule form and as tea, which can be made from either the fresh or dried root.

Vervain—Vervain, another nerve steadier and stimulant, grows wild in the south of France. It is a very powerful tea and has a refreshing taste when honey is added. This herb is also available as a Bach Flower remedy and recommended to workaholics and Type A personalities with high tension levels who need to stop and smell the roses.

Hypericum (St. John's Wort)—Used in ancient Greece for menstrual disorders and in the Middle Ages for anxiety and depression, St. John's Wort (as it is commercially known) is a popular mood elevator touted even by doctors for stabilizing moods and promoting a sense of well-being. A shrub which blossoms on June 24, the birthday of John the Baptist, St. John's Wort is readily available in tablet form but should not be taken in conjunction with Prozac or other clinically prescribed antidepressants without consulting your physician.

Skullcap, used in Native American medicine as a mild sedative and tonic for nervous tension, is available in capsule or tea, and eases tension and induces sleep. Rosemary, utilized for insomnia and depression, is a well-known culinary herb commonly added to stews, casseroles, and salads. It is popular in its herb form or as an essential oil. Other aromatherapy oils which can be used as inhalants, bath oils, or massage oils are lavender, jasmine, sandalwood, and bergamot. Chamomile, an all-round sedative and digestive aid, can also be used in its essential-oil form. Its leaves can be steeped as tea or used to steam the face. Since insomnia is frequently a symptom of depression, herbs and aromatherapy remedies are often interchangeable for treating both ailments. Herbs that heal the digestive tract and/or ease the nervous system include angelica, which stimulates the digestive tract, and balm leaves, which soothe digestion.

DEFEATING INSOMNIA

If you are an insomniac, or simply have difficulty sleeping, try taking a hot bath before bedtime, avoiding stimulants and/or heavy meals after 4:00 P.M., and drinking a glass of warm milk and honey before bedtime. Tryptophan, a mild sedative which produces serotonin, is often recommended to people with sleep disorders. Tryptophan can be taken in supplements or obtained through warm milk, yogurt, turkey, banana, peanut butter, grapefruit, dates, figs, rice, and tuna. Folic acid, inositol, zinc, and vitamins C, D, and E will help you to get a good night's sleep. Tablets containing a combination of calcium and magnesium are also recommended, as are 250 milligrams of magnesium tablets alone. Magnesium can be found in meat, fish, apples, apricots, avocados, bananas, rice, kelp, and garlic.

INCREASE SEROTONIN LEVEL WITH PHYSICAL ACTIVITY

Physical exercise is another method by which serotonin levels are increased, thereby creating a sense of well-being. The Virgoan preoccupation with perfection of mind and body indicates that you probably belong to a fitness club where you can take aerobics classes or utilize treadmills, exercise bicycles, and Stair-Masters to your heart's content. You may even have one or all in your own home. Other physical activities that raise serotonin levels include swimming, running, walking, tennis, or any rigorous activity.

YOGA ASANAS

Since yoga empowers the nervous system while stretching and toning various parts of the body, this ancient Indian philosophy is preferred by many Virgos. Although all yoga positions strengthen the nervous system, some are especially well suited to the lower back and the area surrounding the intestines, which stimulate digestion. For general relaxation, it is important to practice your breathing sitting upright. Rather than the difficult Lotus position, the following Sathasana pose is a modified, cross-legged position which allows you to breathe deeply and comfortably.

SATHASANA

1. Begin by sitting up straight with your spine, head, and neck in a straight, vertical line.
2. Your knees should touch the floor and your ankles should be crossed.
3. Pull your ankles in as close to your body as possible.
4. Rest your wrists on your knees.
5. Keep breathing while sitting as upright as possible.

If you feel that you are supple, you can attempt the Half-Lotus first, followed by the full Lotus position. It is most vital that you proceed at your own pace. Do not attempt to stretch more than your body allows.

HALF-LOTUS

1. Continue to breathe as in the Sathasana position.
2. Take your right leg and place it on your left thigh.
3. Sit upright and keep breathing.

LOTUS

1. With your right leg still on your left thigh, take your left leg and place it on your right thigh.
2. Remain sitting in an upright position and continue to breathe.

DIVERTICULITIS

Diverticulitis results when the diverticula (tiny pouches that can form in the colon) become infected or inflamed. This condition can cause abdominal pain, bloating, nausea, vomiting, chills, and cramping. The severity depends on the extent of the bacterial infection. Because irritable bowel syndrome (IBS) and stomach ulcers cause similar problems, a visit to the doctor is necessary since the diverticula are only revealed through X rays.

Like other ailments, diverticulitis may be treated or prevented by adding dietary fiber to the diet since roughage allows bowel contents to pass easily by keeping stools soft and colon pressure low. Drinking six to eight glasses of water daily also helps.

Processed, or refined, food such as white sugar, flour, and bread as well as coffee, tea, carbonated beverages, and chocolate should be completely eliminated from your diet. Substitute whole-grain breads and cereals, whole-wheat flour that contains wheat bran, and unrefined sugar and honey. (Don't forget that brown sugar is still processed as is most of the honey which is sold in supermarkets.) Unrefined honey is readily available in health food shops. Since Virgos have sensitive intestinal tracts, it may be advantageous to eliminate sweeteners altogether. Try adding cinnamon to coffee (if you must drink it), honey to tea, and raisins, bananas, and/or apples to your cereal. There are many natural, unsweetened fruit juices and jams and jellies available which take the place of sweetened products.

Fruits and vegetables containing roughage include berries, peaches, apples, pears, broccoli, cabbage, cauliflower, spinach, asparagus, squash, and carrots. Wash apples, pears, peaches, or potatoes thoroughly so you can eat the skins, which provide roughage, vitamins, and minerals. Dried beans, barley, and bran are also excellent high-fiber foods.

Products such as Citrucel or Metamucil taken once a day provide about 4 to 6 grams of fiber* when mixed in an 8-ounce glass of water. In most cases, a high-fiber diet, bed rest, and medication will stop diverticulitis dead in its tracks and prevent a recurrence.

If you think your symptoms may indicate diverticulitis, consult your physician immediately. If not treated, diverticulitis can lead to infections, perforations or tears, blockages, or bleeding.

ULCERS

With Virgo ruling the lower abdominal region and intestinal tract, you may be prone to ulcers. Peptic ulcers are sores or lesions which appear either on the lining of the stomach (gastric ulcers) or in the duodenum, the tube that connects the stomach and intestines (duodenal ulcers), when the stomach produces too much acid and not enough mucus to lubricate the stomach. Smoking, drinking, taking too much aspirin, and, of course, genetic predisposition are all factors in the eruption of ulcers.

Although the bacteria *Helicobacter pylori (H. pylori)* has been identified as the culprit that weakens the stomach's protective lining and causes excess acid, undue emotional and physical stress continually wear down the immune system, making the digestive tract a ripe target for the bacteria invasion.

The most common indications that an ulcer may be on the horizon are bloating, heartburn, and abdominal pain between the breastbone and the navel. Other symptoms include nausea, vomiting, appetite reduction, and weight loss. If you cough up blood or pass a stool that is black or bright red, you may be suf-

---

* *The American Dietetic Association recommends 20 to 35 grams of fiber each day.*

fering from a bleeding ulcer whose symptoms are not always readily apparent. Even if the pain subsides, see a physician immediately if you feel weak as this is symptomatic of a bleeding ulcer.

Other than antibiotics, treatment includes taking antacids, which neutralize the stomach, altering dietary habits, and reducing anxiety. Before it was discovered that ulcers were bacteria induced, bland foods and milk products to coat the stomach were recommended. Although it temporarily lines the stomach, milk actually stimulates stomach acid production in the long run, thereby aggravating the pain of an existing ulcer. If you have ulcers, or if your stomach reacts to certain foods, eliminate the following irritants and acidic foods from your diet: alcohol, nicotine, white flour and sugar, spicy foods, coffee, tea, cola, and chocolate. Coffee, tea, cola, and chocolate, which contain caffeine, seem to stimulate acid secretion in the stomach and can aggravate the pain of an existing ulcer. Since the stimulation of stomach acid is also attributed to acidic food content, avoid decaffeinated coffee as well.

Although emotional stress is no longer thought to *cause* ulcers, it certainly can increase ulcer pain. High-fiber foods, including fruits, vegetables, and their juices (especially cabbage juice), and whole grains are recommended as is any herbal remedy such as licorice, peppermint, and slippery elm which lines the mucous membranes. Licorice pills inhibit gastric secretions, as do calcium, zinc, and vitamins A, B, C, and E, which can be taken in capsule form or by increasing foods rich in these nutrients. Healing herbs which stimulate digestion are basil, black mustard, chamomile, anise, caraway, coriander, fennel, ginger, goldenseal, marjoram, mustard, nutmeg, parsley, rosemary, and sage.

Mineral Salt

Potassium sulphate (Kali Sulph.), Virgo's mineral salt, helps maintain healthy hair, nails, and skin by transporting oxygen from the blood to the tissue cells, and strengthens the nervous system by rebuilding nerve cells. Foods that contain potassium sulphate include carrots, tomatoes, red beets, lemons, celery, grapefruit, parsnips, apples, whole wheat, rye, and oats.

Treat Digestive Problems with Fragrant Oils

Aromatherapy oils should be utilized to ease nervous tension and provide general relaxation. Select any scent that appeals to your senses. The most popular oils with wonderfully sweet fragrances are rose, jasmine, lavender, and orange blossom.

The following are especially helpful to ease digestive complaints and/or relieve nervous tension. Used as an essential oil or an ingredient in cooked dishes and salads, basil is wonderful for digestion, stimulation, and calming the nerves. Bergamot oil, made from the main ingredient used in Earl Grey tea, is a natural sedative. Caraway stimulates digestion whether eaten as seeds or brewed in tea. Dill prevents vomiting, stops hiccups, and purifies the digestive tract. Fennel seeds, which can be brewed in tea and added to salads, ease stomach inflammation and quiet intestinal disturbances.

When used as massage oil or as an herb in cooking, marjoram relaxes the nerves. To relieve anxiety, depression, and insomnia, try combining marjoram and lemon essential oils. Recognizable to anyone who burns incense or uses its oil for massage, sandalwood oil has a great sedative effect on the nervous system and functions as an antidepressant. Other oils used as bath oils or inhalants to calm the nerves are orange blossom, rose, lavender, and jasmine—all-around beautiful, sweet-smelling scents. Verbena (also known as lemongrass) oil can be safely massaged on the abdomen to aid digestion.

EASE VIRGO TENSION WITH RELAXING MASSAGE

To facilitate digestion and provide relaxation, ask your partner to give you a gentle, relaxing massage. Lie on your back with your eyes closed. Begin by breathing deeply from your diaphragm to relieve tension. Have your partner rub light oil gently over your abdomen. Let his/her hands come down gently, and pause before starting. Then move hands clockwise around the belly in a broad circular motion, gradually increasing the depth of pressure using smaller circles. Continue to breathe slowly and deeply. Complete the massage by resting your partner's hands on your belly with fingers pointing up toward the breastbone. Lie quietly until you feel you are ready to get up and slowly resume your activities.

According to Chinese medicine, excessive thinking and unnecessary worry deplete the spleen (ruled by Virgo), which in turn interferes with digestion and causes fatigue. Worrying also creates lung disturbances, which result in breathlessness, anxiety, and hyperventilation. Applying acupuncture and acupressure to the meridian point corresponding to the spleen can, according to practitioners of Chinese medicine, relieve the aforementioned conditions. Although acupuncture must be practiced by a licensed practitioner, acupressure can be done at home by placing pressure on the point correlating with the spleen. This point is located "on the outer side of the lower leg below the knee joint" (see Fig. 7.1).[7] Unblocking the energy to this area should work wonders for poor digestion, anxiety, headaches, and poor circulation. Even if you do not apply pressure to the precise spots where the acupressure points lie, practicing this exercise will certainly do no harm.

There are other pressure points used in acupressure and shiatsu which can be located with very little knowledge of these disciplines. One that can ease insomnia is located on the neck about one inch below the bottom of the ear lobe. Press hard against this point with your index finger for about fifteen to twenty seconds on one side of the neck and repeat the same motion on the other side.

AYURVEDA

Due to nervousness, irritability, and too much mental activity, Virgos can be, like Geminis, classified as Vata dosha. Your digestive system is easily upset and especially sensitive to spicy and gaseous foods. Vata is characterized by restlessness, insomnia, anxiety, fatigue, and depression. Vata types place excessive demands on themselves and others, creating an atmosphere of constant pressure. To alter these habits, you must begin by getting a sufficient amount of rest. The moment you feel you have reached your capacity physically and mentally, stop and take a break.

Besides mastering relaxation techniques, it is important that Vata types change their eating habits. Learn to eat slowly and wait at least one hour after meals before participating in physical activity. Add salty, sour, and sweet foods (see Appendix II) to your diet. Milk, stews, warm soups, hot cereals, and freshly baked, warm bread* are all soothing for your body type. Begin the day with a substantial breakfast of cream of rice or wheat.

---

* *The bread can be either white bread or wheat bread. The important element here is that it is warm.*

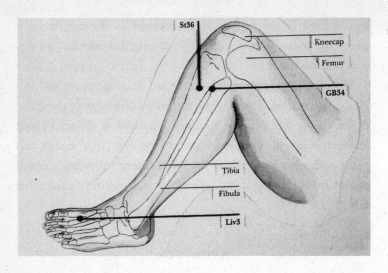

FIGURE 7.1 SPLEEN ACUPRESSURE POINT

Get into the habit of drinking warm herbal tea throughout the day as you may find yourself getting cold easily. Classified as pungent, ginger stimulates digestion and can be used as a condiment in cooking or as a tea. Other spices that are digestive aids include cinnamon, fennel, and cardamom. When you feel the signs of anxiety or nervousness approaching, prepare a hot cup of tea or cream of vegetable soup. Warm grains like lentils, pasta, and rice with melted butter added are also recommended for Vata types.

GEM AND COLOR THERAPY

If you were born between August 23 and August 31, your birthstone is the peridot, a semiprecious stone; if you were born between September 1 and September 20, your gemstone is the sapphire, a beautiful blue semiprecious stone. Other gems associated with Virgo are agate, sardonyx, marble, and jasper. Metals are nickel, copper, and quicksilver, the chemical name for mercury (Mercury is Virgo's ruling planet). Virgo colors are blue and gray.

Chapter 8

Libra the Scales

Lazy and Indulgent
but Can Vanity Conquer All?

LIBRA THE SCALES
(SEPTEMBER 21–OCTOBER 22)
RULING PLANET: Venus
ELEMENT: Air
MODALITY: Cardinal

Positive Libra traits and concepts are artistic, harmonious, diplomatic, fair-minded, personable, social, considerate, refined, aesthetic, intellectual, loving, truthful, impartial, affable, cooperative, sympathetic, graceful, charming, creative, idealistic, gentle, rational, and even-tempered.

Negative Libra traits and concepts are indecisive, manipulative, lazy, gluttonous, low self-esteem, follows the crowd, dishonest, critical, indulgent, unemotional, detached, hedonistic, dominating, dependent, superficial, and unrealistic.

Parts of the body ruled by Libra include the kidneys, diaphragm, pancreas, adrenal glands, abdomen, and lower back. Your ruling planet, Venus, governs the eyes and the skin. Ailments include acne, skin rash (psoriasis), oily skin, dermatitis, kidney stones, diabetes, eating disorders, obesity, edema, alcohol and drug addiction, and hypoglycemia.

Professions which appeal to the Libran sense of aesthetics, harmony, and beauty as well as their love of people, politics and socializing include artist, writer, musician, fashion consultant, beautician, graphic designer, interior decorator, fashion model, politician, therapist, social worker, diplomat, judge, mediator, advertising, human resources, receptionist, and counselor.

LIBRA THE SCALES:
COOPERATION—KEY TO THE LIBRAN SUCCESS

Ruled by Venus, planet of love and beauty, sensual and charming Librans are gentle, artistic, yet obsessed with being in love, having a partner, and never being alone. Cooperative, tactful, and proud of your ability to share, you are distinctly aware that "two heads are better than one." You have the ability to maintain all types of relationships and associations by practicing the art of compromise better than any other sign.

Classified as a cardinal air sign, Libra, symbolized by the scales of justice, has clarity of vision, remarkable objectivity, and sound reasoning ability. A superb mediator who sees both sides of an issue, you are the first to be called upon for impartial opinions, to clarify situations, or to settle disputes. Your unique ability to remain calm and focused always provides comfort and assistance in the midst of a personal or professional crisis.

Although it may appear contradictory for a sign so relationship-oriented to appear aloof and even detached, it must be remembered that Libra, an air sign, and the only one represented by an inanimate object, is motivated neither by passion nor emotions but by a need for companionship, communication, and approval from others.

Rational and even-tempered, you are endowed with great finesse and social skills and will remain socially acceptable by suppressing undesirable emotions (i.e., fear, anger, hostility). When confronted with stress, however, your bottled-up reticence and politeness can suddenly explode, bringing on the very negativity you hoped to avoid.

A case in point occurred at a party I attended. A charming and outgoing Libran friend, not wishing to offend his host and hostess, agreed to stay for dinner against his better judgment—his exhaustion should have precipitated an early departure. Ironically, his inability to relax and enjoy the evening (made obvious by continual glances at his watch) transformed him into a tense, unresponsive guest whose early exit would have, in the long run, been more considerate.

This reaction is symptomatic of a significant Libran trait—the tendency to act in accordance with another's expectation in order to gain respect, love, and/or admiration. As a result, you rarely express an opinion or make a decision until you are certain that at least one other person shares your views. While you are praised by some for being kind, sensitive, and considerate, you infuriate others by remaining neutral and refusing to take a stand.

While your placidity and ease may give the impression of self-assurance, Librans are, in actuality, often plagued with enormous self-doubt. Rather than continually seeking advice and approval, why not rely on your own sound judgment and intuition? A supportive and caring partner who can help strengthen your self-esteem may provide the incentive to focus on the future and the stamina necessary to forge ahead.

PHYSIOGNOMY AND BODY TYPE

The Libra type is often characterized by soft hair, calm eyes, slightly pointed nose, well-formed mouth, wide lips, and an elegant neck. Your features are usually refined, giving a fragile and delicate appearance. What sets you apart is that gleam in your eye, a flirtatious manner, and an unabashed facility for making friends.

Libra rules the kidneys, abdomen, diaphragm, adrenal glands, and lower back, while its governing planet, Venus, rules the skin and the eyes. Your lethargic nature, lack of exercise, love of rich foods, and bon vivant lifestyle accompanied by excessive habits contribute to easy weight gain. The bad news is that you must exert a great deal of effort in the struggle to develop good eating habits and weave physical exercise into your daily routine. On a positive note, the desire to be praised and preoccupation with appearance may motivate you to stay on the straight and narrow, preventing increased poundage. Although Librans are strongly influenced by the opinions of others, try to ignore celluloid images and rely on your own intuition. Remember that beauty is truly skin deep and how you feel inside is what really counts.

AILMENTS AFFECTING YOUR KIDNEYS

When consumption of rich foods, an abundance of sweets, and too much alcohol is not offset by regular physical activity, the kidneys may be forced to work overtime to eliminate excess fat, water, and impurities from the body. The kidneys, two bean-shaped organs located below the ribs toward the middle of the back, regulate the process of elimination by converting excess water and wastes from the blood into urine. Early warning signs that the kidneys are not functioning optimally appear when toxins are released not through elimination but in the form of mild acne, profuse sweating, and water ringlets below the eyes. The most obvious sign is the onset of edema, that is, swelling of the ankles, knees, and/or fingers due to water retention. If you notice that this is occurring, be certain to elevate your legs, and avoid wearing tight shoes or stockings. In extreme cases, renal malfunction (which can also be the result of congenital weakness) contributes to hypoglycemia, diabetes, gallstones, liver problems, and the production of excruciatingly painful kidney stones.

Kidney stones are formed when salt and minerals separate from urine, build up on the inner surfaces of the kidney, and crystallize. If the crystals are tiny, they will travel through the urinary tract and pass out of the body unnoticed. Once the stone is passed, it would be extremely helpful to have it analyzed to see if it is, like the majority of stones, calcium based. If so, cut down on the following calcium-rich foods: apples, asparagus, beer, beans, beets, berries, broccoli, cheese, grapes, ice cream, milk, oranges, parsley, peanut butter, pineapples, spinach, tea, turnips, and yogurt. If the stone is too large and cannot be expelled, it will cause agonizing pain in the lower back. The only alternative is medication to help pass the stone or having it removed either surgically or through noninvasive procedures such as laser or ultrasound treatment.

But by far the most important preventive measure is drinking six to eight glasses of water daily. Water flushes the kidneys of excess fat and waste, which in turn prevents the crystallization of salt and minerals. Protein increases the amount of uric acid, calcium, and phosphorus in the urine, thereby aiding the manufacture of stones. Watch the intake of meat, fish, poultry, and cheese. Avoid chocolate, coffee, cola and other caffeinated products. Don't season food with salt or eat salty snacks like potato chips and pretzels. Avoid pickled foods and food preservatives containing sodium nitrite.

Green and yellow fruits and vegetables such as sweet potatoes, pumpkin, squash, cantaloupe, and apricots are rich in vitamin A, which helps line the urinary tract, hampering the formation of stones. Do not take more than the RDA (recommended dietary allowance) of five thousand vitamin A units, and remember that supplements should not be taken without professional advice since large amounts can be harmful.

High-fiber foods like oat bran are essential for Librans, who must constantly cleanse and purify their systems. Other foods that act as natural diuretics include radishes, celery, cucumber, parsley, oats, asparagus, kidney beans, and carrots. Be careful not to eat too many fruits and vegetables as they can create a surplus of gas in an already sensitive system.

The consumption of cranberry juice has been touted by some as a means to ward off kidney stone production, but it is doubtful that a sufficient amount can be consumed to make the urine acidic enough. (Also, most cranberry juice is sweetened, which somewhat lessens its effects.) If you find the taste of this refreshing, healthy beverage pleasing, however, that is a good enough reason to drink it.

Herbs and plants that stimulate the kidneys, thereby purifying the body of toxins, are bilberry, borage, parsley, horseradish, and thyme. Senna and pennyroyal, strong herbal diuretics taken in tea or powder form, certainly aid in activating the kidneys and cleansing the system but should only be taken in extremely small doses. Ingesting an excessive amount can cause stomach contractions and overtax the kidneys, causing potential long-term damage. It is imperative to heed the instructions on the label and, if you have had digestive problems, senna or pennyroyal should not be taken until your physician has been consulted. Neither of these herbs should be taken by pregnant women, as both can cause contractions which may result in miscarriage. Exercise caution with all over-the-counter diuretics since overuse can result in kidney damage.

ADULT ACNE

The skin and the kidneys come under the auspices of Venus, Libra's ruling planet. Excess oils and toxins not flushed out by the kidneys may be released through the sebaceous glands and skin as perspiration and acne, respectively. Acne is an umbrella term for the noninflamed and inflamed lesions (commonly called pimples) that appear on the chin, nose, and cheeks—the most oily parts of the face—when the skin is clogged with excess oil. Especially prevalent among adolescents and premenstrual women, whose hormones produce an overage of oil, this condition can usually be kept under control if the pores are deep-cleansed. Acne can range from a few pimples here and there to an advanced infection which can itch, burn, and be especially unsightly. While stress, sunlight, and hereditary factors will aggravate these breakouts, it has long been erroneously believed that greasy and oily foods cause the sebaceous glands to overact. Because the skin is especially sensitive and your nervous system so fragile, it is important not to touch, scratch, or pick at these blemishes, or overload yourself with emotional stress.

Frequently mistaken for acne, rosacea, a chronic adult skin

condition, is caused mainly by genetic factors. Characterized by red spots, inflamed, raised blemishes, or pustules (pus-filled blemishes), the breakout is confined to the center of the face. Avoid anything which causes a flush such as alcohol, spices, or very hot water. Do not use topical products manufactured for acne as they can worsen this ailment. Bill Clinton's nose and cheeks are examples of the appearance of rosacea. He is a Leo Sun sign, but at his precise time of birth, Venus, Mars, Neptune, and his ascendant were all placed in the sign of Libra—a unique example of how the zodiacal signs affect health beyond the sign of your Sun.

Since looking your best is vital to your self-esteem, choose makeup that contains no oil, chemicals, or other skin irritants so as not to clog your pores even more. Cleanse your face thoroughly with chemical-free, clear soap that does not irritate the skin and will rid it of dirt, makeup, and excess oil. Herbal cleansers made with almonds and cucumbers are highly recommended. If you must use a commercial cleanser, buy only those which are gentle. Do not under any circumstances go to bed without removing makeup. Your skin is the first line of defense, and must be clean in order for it to breathe, retain moisture, and keep irritants out. On the other hand, be careful not to overcleanse. Too much scrubbing can result in redness, rashes, or dermatitis—a condition which may also be caused by an allergic reaction. The best method is simply to wash your face with lukewarm water several times a day for deep cleansing. Once the pores have been opened, use a mild astringent after washing to close them and prevent dirt from seeping in.

FACIAL MASSAGE

Since Librans are creatures of comfort, luxury, and sensual pleasures, there is probably nothing more enjoyable than being pampered and massaged. Although your entire body responds to the sensation of touch, your face will especially reap the benefits of massage, which increases blood supply, stimulates skin function, improves muscle tone, and may even clear up pimples or acne. Massage helps relieve facial tension and will make you look and feel more relaxed and years younger. You can either give yourself a facial massage or have your partner do it for you. If you opt for the latter, be sure to promise your partner one in return. It is especially gratifying if the person applying the massage sits across from the receiver so there is eye contact. If this makes you uncomfortable, then the person receiving the massage should simply sit in front of the masseur or masseuse.

The following variations outline the best procedure for massaging the face. You can perform the entire series at one sitting or focus on a few of the movements each time you give, or are given, a massage.

1. Begin by pulling your hair back using a coated rubber band, headband, or scarf so that the massage oil does not touch your scalp.
2. Rubbing just a slight amount of massage oil into your fingers, guide them up the sides of your face with gentle strokes starting from the jawline and moving slowly up to the forehead. Repeat this motion several times until your face starts feeling relaxed.
3. Pat your forehead with the palms of your hands moving from your eyebrows up to the point where your hairline begins. This movement should be smooth and even.

4. Reverse the motion by guiding your fingers from the hairline downward and then across the eyebrows.

5. Rest your palms on your forehead for a few seconds. Then move your palms from the center of your forehead outward toward your ear lobes. Repeat this movement several times.

6. With your index and middle finger, massage your temples gently yet firmly with circular motions for several minutes.

7. Glide your fingers over your eyebrow slowly and gently using the thumb and index finger. If you use your thumb, you will be applying slightly more pressure than with the other fingers. Close your eyelids. Use either your ring finger or the palms of your hands to stroke your eyelids from corner to corner and from top to bottom. Repeat these movements three to five times.

8. Then gently move your thumbs down your nose and around the tip of the nostrils, making sure you do not press too hard.

9. Move your first two fingers along your cheekbone, down the side of your face, to your chin, and down along your neck. Making sure your hands are still somewhat damp from massage oil, reverse the motion and bring your hands up from your neck to the chin and upward along the cheeks. Repeat these two movements three times.

10. End this relaxing massage by stroking your forehead, then patting it gently, and finally resting your palms over your eyes with your fingers directed upward toward the forehead.[8]

HEED THE WARNING SIGNS OF DIABETES

If there is a history of diabetes (short for diabetes mellitus) in your family, you may already have a gene which predisposes you to this chronic disease presently affecting 16 million American adults and children. Although it is the fourth leading cause of death in the United States, diabetes continues to go undetected by many who have it. Diabetes falls into two categories:

1. Type I-insulin dependent or juvenile diabetes occurs when the pancreas, governed by Libra, ceases to produce the hormone insulin.
2. Type II-non-insulin dependent diabetes results when insulin is underproduced, or when the body fails to properly utilize the insulin manufactured by the pancreas.

In both instances, glucose remains in the blood and is, therefore, unable to pass on to the body's cells. As a result, the high levels of blood sugar can damage nerves and kidneys, cause blindness, increase the risk of heart disease and stroke, and generally damage the immune system, slowing up the body's healing process. About 90 percent of all diabetics fall into the Type II category, which can be controlled through diet, exercise, and medication without the necessity of insulin injections, required in the case of Type I diabetes.

While genetic proclivity does not guarantee that you will succumb to this illness, it does mean that if diabetes runs in your family, you must be more careful than most about your diet. Aside from heredity factors, you may be a candidate for this disease if you are overweight, inactive, have high blood pressure or high cholesterol, had diabetes during pregnancy, or had a baby over nine pounds. Although any Sun sign may be genetically prone to this ailment, your sedentary habits and the tendency toward food and alcohol excess make you especially vulnerable to diabetes later in life. The warning signs include extreme thirst, blurry vision, frequent urination, unusual fatigue, unexplained weight loss, recurring skin, gum, or bladder infections that heal slowly, and tingling or numbness in the hands and feet. If you suffer from several of these, see your physician immediately.

Fortunately, diabetes can often be controlled or even averted altogether through regulated eating habits and exercise plans. Although a healthy diet and physical exercise are a universal panacea for feeling good no matter what your sign, Libras especially benefit since many of their ailments are directly related to excessive habits. Blood-sugar levels and blood pressure can be kept as close to normal as possible by maintaining a low-fat diet, eliminating nicotine, exercising regularly, limiting alcohol, and eating smaller meals more frequently. It is recommended that about 50 percent of caloric intake be obtained from carbohydrates, which are either simple (sugars) or complex (starches), with 12 to 20 percent of caloric intake obtained from protein. Whole-wheat products, barley, oats, fruit, and legumes are the best sources of fiber. Because fiber is filling, eating reasonable amounts to satisfy your hunger will make weight control simpler.

There are supplements on the market that can help maintain normal blood-sugar levels and keep blood pressure under control, but should not be taken unless prescribed by a professional. Among these are chromium G.T.F., niacin, vitamin C, zinc, magnesium, vitamin B_6, inositol (vitamin B), thiamine (B_1), garlic, and acidophilus. Over-the-counter supplements should always be checked for warnings directed to diabetics.

If you are diabetic, the safest, least stressful, and most effective exercise is walking briskly. Since nerve damage (neuropathy), a side effect of the disease, decreases the sensation of pain, diabetics are often unaware that they have injured their feet, and a little sore can potentially become gangrenous. Feet must be kept dry and clean and should be inspected several times a day to see if there are any cuts, bruises, blisters, swelling, or infection.

If you are diabetic or think you may be leaning in that direction, be certain to get a thorough blood workup once a year so that your physician can detect changes in your blood-sugar level. There are over-the-counter blood-glucose testing kits which can help you keep tabs on blood-sugar levels when used accurately. Because stress can make blood sugar go haywire, visualization exercises and relaxation techniques which focus on controlled breathing can also help. Hypoglycemia occurs when blood-sugar levels drop too low, causing headaches, confusion, or, at the most extreme, unconsciousness, which requires immediate medical attention.

Hyperglycemia, on the other hand, occurs when blood sugar levels rise too high. Mild symptoms are frequent urination, increased appetite, thirst, blurry vision, or dizziness. Severe symptoms are loss of appetite, stomach cramps, nausea, vomiting, dehydration, fatigue, and rapid breathing. If these occur, go to the emergency room at once.

Love Is the Answer

Since Libra is ruled by Venus, being alone is excruciating and the stress it causes can be almost intolerable. There is often a tendency to alleviate the anxiety, tension, and loneliness with food, alcohol, and/or drugs. Social Libra needs a supportive companion—one who will raise your spirits when you are feeling down, relieve despair, offer general support, and provide sensual pleasure—a healthy substitute for food, alcohol, or drugs. With a partner, you are more likely to engage in moderate living habits, and even learn to exercise together (since you hate doing this on your own).

On the other hand, you must be cautious that you do not enter into codependent relationships, that is, preserving a relationship at all costs to avoid being alone. Taken to the extreme, you may even overlook your partner's addictions or problems in order to be needed. Since Librans thrive on sharing confidences, and are often counselors or therapists themselves, drop-in groups where attendees either speak out or listen may be appealing. Many drop-in groups have twelve-step programs which involve a sponsor—a recovering confidante who will help you change your lifestyle and guide you through the recovery process to avoid a relapse. Alanon is a twelve-step program devoted to helping family members and partners of those with addictive behavior patterns ranging from alcoholism to drug addiction to gambling. If you are in a relationship with someone who exhibits self-destructive behavior, or if you are "enabling" your partner, that is, tolerating or even encouraging the addiction so you will be needed, then Alanon is the support group for you. If group dynamics do not suit you, seek one-on-one counseling to help manage stress and improve your coping skills.

Since you love the creative arts but dislike doing anything on your own, combining exercise with social activities may be the incentive you need. Opt for a dance, aerobics, or yoga class rather than solitary activities like swimming, running, walking, or bicycling. Try ballroom dancing or figure skating—both creative and fun. Visit a health spa that offers herbal wraps, massages, saunas, and swimming as well as yoga and aerobics classes, which combine physical activity with the desire to look and feel good.

YOGA POSITIONS

Libran's rulership over the lower part of the body combined with a sedentary, lethargic lifestyle may lead to bad posture and lower back pain. Acupressure and acupuncture work wonders to ease discomfort of lower back pain by circulating energy and increasing vitality. In addition to the Plow Pose (the yoga position outlined in Chapter 6), the Cobra is a very popular and easy asana to master which elongates and strengthens the lower back, stretches the abdominal muscles, and can help relieve uterine and ovarian problems.

COBRA POSE (FIG 8.1)

1. Lie facedown on your stomach.
2. Bring your feet together with your hands directly under your shoulders and fingers pointing forward. Slightly elongate the spine to prevent your lower back from crunching up.
3. On the inhalation, lift and expand the chest forward as you press down with your hands. Keep your elbows close to the body and continue to widen and lengthen your spine. Move your shoulders downward and away from your ears to free the neck and head. Allow the upper back to widen and elongate.
4. Hold for a few breaths, exhale, then slowly come down.
5. Repeat the pose one to three times. Continue to breathe normally keeping the spine extended. Let the body completely relax.

SHOULDER STAND (FIG 8.2)

The Sarvangasana, or Shoulder Stand, is simpler than the head stand and will reverse the flow of gravity, allowing tension to be drawn from the abdomen.

1. Lie flat on your back with legs outstretched.
2. Bend your legs and slowly bring the knees backward over your chest.

3. Using elbows and backs of upper arms, support your lower back with the palms of your hands with thumbs outspread.
4. Elbows should not be wider than the shoulders.
5. Raise trunk to the vertical position.
6. Straighten legs so that they form a vertical line.
7. Keep your chest against your chin, and breathe freely.

AYURVEDA

Since Venus is classified as a Kapha planet, Libra, like Taurus and Cancer, fits the profile of this slow, lethargic, and very cold dosha. Although wonderfully creative and cooperative to the point of never reaching a decision without the approval of others, you have difficulty directing your energies toward a clear goal. Easily distracted, you often find reasons why you are incapable of bringing projects to fruition, and finishing what you begin.

Librans, like yourself, are characterized by enjoyment of sensual pleasures, laziness, and indulgent behavior, which Ayurvedic practitioners attribute, in part, to lack of exercise and consumption of too many sweet and salty foods. It is to your advantage to eat food which is warm, light, and dry with a minimum of butter, oil, and sugar. Pungent, bitter, and astringent food will stimulate your digestion and help you to control your weight. Since you may have a tendency to retain water, abstain from flavoring your food with salt. Vegetables should be grilled and baked rather than boiled. If you think of yourself as light, or floating in air, you will be attracted to lightly cooked foods, as well as raw fruits and vegetables. Spicy, or pungent, foods such as onions, garlic, and ginger stimulate digestion and will keep your body warm, while bitter and astringent foods can help reduce your appetite. (See Appendix II.)

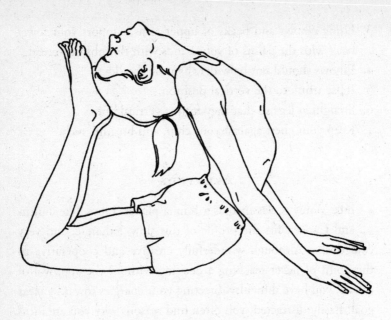

FIGURE 8.1 COBRA POSE

AROMATHERAPY AND ESSENTIAL OILS

Librans are especially receptive to scents with an aromatic bouquet which help to alleviate skin discomforts. Popular, sweet-smelling jasmine is often used in the form of incense, cologne, bath oil, or hot, aromatic tea. Jasmine oil is recommended for dry skin, and may also be rubbed on the abdomen to ease stomachaches or menstrual cramps. Lemongrass oil does wonders for acne and other oily skin conditions, as does bergamot when steam from the tea's steeped leaves envelops the face. To ease eczema, dermatitis, and sagging, sluggish skin, massage geranium oil into the face and neck. Used in a bath or rubbed onto

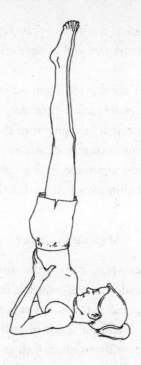

FIGURE 8.2 SHOULDER STAND

the neck and shoulders, it also alleviates nervous tension and anxiety. Lavender oil relieves skin irritations and acne when used to massage the face, or lightly dabbed on the affected areas as a freshener. If your skin is oily, combine lemon, lavender, bergamot, juniper, or ylang-ylang with witch hazel. If acne is the problem, add lemongrass, lavender, juniper, or chamomile to distilled or mineral water. If your skin is hypersensitive, add chamomile, orange blossom, jasmine, or rose to orange flower water. To ease boils, dermatitis, eczema, and rashes, add chamomile oil to a small cotton compress saturated in hot water. Apply it to the afflicted area and remove once the compress has cooled.

Regardless of the combination you select, two drops of aromatherapy oil will usually suffice. After deep-cleansing your face, add the essential oil which best suits your skin texture to a small piece of cloth or damp cotton wool. Afterward, wipe your entire face and neck with the compress, paying special attention to the creases around your chin where oil tends to congregate.

MINERAL SALT

Sodium phosphate (Nat. Phos.), the mineral salt associated with Libra, is needed to maintain the acid and alkaline balance. It also helps equalize the body's water balance to prevent bloating and water retention. Lack of sodium phosphate may lead to heartburn, poor digestion, as well as poor functioning of the kidneys and liver. Sodium phosphate is present in watercress, carrots, spinach, peas, celery, beets, yellow corn, strawberries, apples, raisins, figs, almonds, rice, and wheat.

GEMS AND COLOR THERAPY

If you were born between September 21 and September 30, your birthstone is the sapphire, a blue or white precious stone. If you were born between October 1 and October 22, your birthstone is the opal, a beautiful bluish-white semiprecious stone. Since its colors are white and green, Libra's stones include diamonds, zircon (imitation diamonds), white quartz, and alabaster as well as emerald, tourmaline, and jade, which are green. To improve your relationships and bring love into your life, these gemstones must touch the skin and be set in white gold, the metal associated with Venus, Libra's ruling planet. Since green and white are Libran colors, get off the sofa and head for the nearest park where you can walk, bicycle, and commune with nature as often as possible. If you are lucky enough to live outside a city, spend time outdoors, where grass and trees abound.

Chapter 9

Scorpio the Scorpion

Too Much Control
Is Detrimental to Your Health

♏

SCORPIO THE SCORPION
(OCTOBER 23–NOVEMBER 22)
RULING PLANET: Pluto (coruler Mars)
ELEMENT: Water
MODALITY: Fixed

Positive Scorpio traits and concepts are single-minded, exciting, ambitious, serious, intense, passionate, sexual, magnetic, persevering, transformative, emotional, enterprising, ingenious, intuitive, high-energy, financially adept, and loyal.

Negative Scorpio traits and concepts are self-destructive, unforgiving, promiscuous, surreptitious, manipulative, jealous, hedonistic, selfish, power-hungry, possessive, vengeful, mean-spirited, obstinate, inflexible, domineering, and intractable.

Parts of the body ruled by Scorpio include the colon, bladder, prostate gland, reproductive organs, genitals, and rectum. Your ruling planet, Pluto, governs the endocrine system.

Ailments include hemorrhoids, sexually transmitted diseases, cystitis, urinary tract infections, bowel disorders, hernia, bladder infections, constipation, and, in the extreme, prostate and ovarian difficulties.

Professions which bring out Scorpio's need for financial risk taking, adventure, challenges, competition, research, and physical activity include researcher, scientist, engineer, doctor, psychologist, mystery writer, filmmaker, contractor, mathematician, photographer, detective, artist, stockbroker, financial consultant, military personnel, physicist, and athlete.

SCORPIO THE SCORPION:
OUT OF THE DARKNESS AND INTO THE LIGHT

A fixed water sign, and the eighth of the zodiac, Scorpio is passionate, intense, highly creative, yet manipulative, domineering, and controlling. Not unlike your symbol, the venomous scorpion, you can attack at a moment's notice if you feel an injustice has been perpetrated or you have been wronged. You tend to see life as a war with distinctly defined battle zones—people are either for you or against you. An absolute extremist, you range from being overly sensitive and defensive to becoming vindictive and vengeful in a split second.

Ardent, sexual, and highly charged, you have an intensity which is unlike that of any other sign. An amazing workaholic with an immense capacity for taking charge, you have the stamina to accomplish in one day what others couldn't do in a week. Boundless energy, personal magnetism, and a steely discipline are the tools of the trade to attain success—yet you often sacrifice personal relationships along the way. Once your goals are set in motion, you are relentless, even ruthless, in pursuit of them.

With Pluto, Greco-Roman lord of the underworld, as your ruling planet, you are capable of great emotional extremes which range from immeasurable ecstasy to dark moments of deep depression. An avid conversationalist and intent listener in comfortable surroundings, you are apprehensive, introverted, and even cold when thrust into an unfamiliar milieu. Once you let your guard down, an enthusiastic and warm personality is instantly revealed. Until that moment of familiarity arrives, however, it's anyone's guess whether Dr. Jekyll or Mr. Hyde will emerge.

You find it difficult to express sadness, anger, trepidation, or even love, for fear that your overwhelming emotions may force you to lose control. Once your buttons are pushed, however, suppressed feelings eventually do surface and, like a burst dam, overpower your rational mind and sound judgment. Try to verbalize what you are feeling without worrying about the reactions of others. Until you do, you will continue to be caught up in the same vicious circle.

Learning to confront problems by discussing them openly can prevent unnecessary stress, phobias, and, more extreme, paranoia. Since you are compulsive, even obsessive, seek emotional release through your favorite activities—artistry, athletics, and financial wheeling and dealing. With Scorpio ruling the sexual organs, you may also find release through intimate relationships, though jealousy and insecurity often threaten the love you share.

Don't ever rest on your laurels. Use your concentration and resourcefulness to find new worlds to conquer and projects into which you can sink your teeth. Do be realistic about your true capabilities. If you find you cannot live up to your impossibly high standards and unrealistic expectations, don't punish yourself by engaging in self-destructive behavior, including compulsive gambling, chronic overeating, alcoholism, or drug addiction. When you experience disappointment, try to ward off your tendency toward dark moods and potential long-term depression. Get off the couch, lace up your sneakers, and try walking or running it off. Walking briskly or running for about twenty-five minutes will release endorphins and help you relax. If you really find that you cannot kick those dark moods and you find yourself spending more and more time alone, force yourself to call someone you trust or see a therapist. (See Chapter 7 for depression tips.)

PHYSIOGNOMY AND BODY TYPE

Serious and determined, Scorpios can be recognized by an intense, piercing look so seething and, at times, intimidating that others may avoid eye contact to hide their discomfort. You are easily identifiable by a low forehead, bushy eyebrows, hook nose, and deep-set eyes—your most distinguishing characteristic. At times, you convey calmness and even serenity. But there is usually a storm brewing below. Back problems, a stiff neck, muscle tears, and torn ligaments are common problems for Scorpios, who tend to push beyond the limit. (See Chapter 6 for yoga and stretching exercises which can elongate the spine.)

Scorpios have always utilized intense activity as a way to stay in shape and release both physical and emotional tension. Due to a penchant for pushing yourself to the limit, you are probably attracted to strenuous activities which provide excitement and challenge, including downhill skiing, scuba diving, aquatic sports, and bungee jumping. A competitive nature and the need to constantly challenge your abilities and test your limits also fares well in tennis, squash, boxing, or even race-car driving. While most of these activities provide a fabulous workout, don't go overboard if you have passed your fortieth birthday. Since you thrive on competition, team sports like basketball, soccer, and football will provide a vigorous workout. Remember to balance your need to shine with the demands of being a team player.

After you have pushed yourself to your limit to release aggression, relax your muscles so that physical tension will be eased and chronic pains will be lessened. You may rebel against yoga and stretching exercises, but they will, in the long run, revitalize and relax a tension-ridden body.

MASSAGE THERAPY

Having your body gently and lovingly stroked is a wonderful panacea for easing rigidity and pent-up anger. Once you learn to relax, relationships and communication will be somewhat easier. Regular massages by a professional, or your partner, will relieve tenseness and even prevent an outburst when tension appears to be approaching explosive levels. Swedish massage is a very gentle form of touch, both uplifting and therapeutic without the risk of injury to vulnerable body parts.

This form of massage may, however, not be powerful or therapeutic enough to iron out the kinks. Shiatsu, acupressure, deep-tissue massage, or even Rolfing are techniques whereby concentrated, sometimes extremely uncomfortable pressure is applied to certain points on the body to help release emotional pain and blocked tension. These methods require the expertise of a professional since the massage can be ineffective or even damaging if applied to the wrong place with the incorrect amount of pressure. Infant massage, a series of gentle manipulative techniques designed for children, should be introduced to Scorpio children early on as they are certain to exhibit their hallmark obstinacy and inflexibility at a young age.

Other than relaxation techniques, yoga, deep massage, and even sexual release (which is often Scorpios' outlet), the best remedy for Scorpionic rigidity is expressing yourself clearly and verbalizing emotions. It is also the most difficult. If you are having communication or intimacy problems with your partner, consider attending couples' counseling sessions. Of course, this will not be an easy task given your reticence. Then again, Scorpios usually love challenges.

CONSTIPATION

Scorpios' tendency to overwork keeps them on the go for hours without exercising the bowels. While self-control may serve you well in certain situations, it can become a long-term health problem if you allow too much time to elapse between nature's calls. Since physical requirements differ from one person to the next, the need to go to the bathroom varies, despite the fact that laxative advertisements would have you believe that a daily bowel movement is a must for good health. If more than three days pass without a bowel movement, however, the intestinal contents may harden, making it painful for stools to pass.

A principal cause of constipation is a diet high in animal fats (meats, dairy products, eggs) and refined sugar (rich desserts and other sweets), but low in fiber (vegetables, fruits, whole grains). For most people, dietary and lifestyle improvements will decrease the chances of constipation. A well-balanced diet that includes fiber-rich foods, such as unprocessed bran, whole-grain breads, and fresh fruits and vegetables is recommended. Drinking plenty of fluids and exercising regularly will help to stimulate intestinal activity.

If constipation persists and stools do not pass easily due to improper diet and irregular toilet habits, hemorrhoids, the veins in and around the anus, will swell. Lifting heavy objects, exercising strenuously, and straining to eliminate exacerbates the condition, which can, in the extreme, lead to bleeding and excruciating pain. To avoid chronic constipation, and ultimately hemorrhoids, the following dietary and lifestyle changes are suggested:

1. Eat a well-balanced diet rich in high-fiber foods such as raw fruit (including apples, peaches, raspberries, and tangerines), vegetables (including acorn squash, broccoli, brussels sprouts, cabbage, carrots, cauliflower, spinach, and zucchini), black-eyed peas, kidney beans, lima beans, whole-grain cereal, and whole-wheat or seven-grain bread.

2. Start each morning with a tablespoon of unprocessed bran or another high-fiber cereal to initiate bowel movements. Continue to eat three or four tablespoons throughout the day, adding it to salads, soups, and sandwiches, and you will begin to feel lighter and less bloated. Avoid high-fat breakfasts like bacon and eggs, which clog the bowels.

3. Limit foods that have little or no fiber, including animal fat (meats, dairy products, eggs), refined sugar and flour, salty snacks, and processed foods, which interfere with the process of elimination.

4. A minimum of six to eight glasses of fluids—preferably water—should become part of the daily routine, as they flush the bowels. Try herbal tea (especially ginger), clear soup, and fruit and vegetable juice. Ginseng, which is available in tea, powder, capsule, or tonic form, often works wonders—stimulates the appetite, digestion, and bowels. It is also a known

aphrodisiac, which should appeal to Scorpios. Avoid alcohol, and coffee and other caffeinated beverages.

5. Like Cancer and Pisces, the other water signs, Scorpios retain water and, as such, should make a concerted effort to reduce their salt intake (see Chapter 6 for hints). Substitute condiments like black pepper and garlic, or adjust your taste buds by eating blander foods. Other foods containing sodium that should be avoided include onion salt, celery salt, garlic salt, and soy sauce. Be sure to check the labels of canned, frozen, and low-fat foods, since they usually contain an overabundance of sodium preservatives. Your best bet is abstaining from packaged low-fat foods altogether in favor of fruits and vegetables, whole-grain breads, pasta, and broiled or grilled meat, poultry, and fish. Avoid naturally salted food such as cheese, smoked or cured meat, pickles, sauerkraut, sardines, and anchovies.

6. Exercise regularly. Activity keeps the bowels working and combats constipation by moving food through the system at a faster pace. A twenty- to thirty-minute brisk walk daily will do the trick. Avoid straining, lifting heavy objects, wearing tight clothing, and other movements which will put pressure on the bowels.

7. Never ignore the urge to relieve yourself.

8. Give yourself a mental suggestion to go to the bathroom after each meal, thereby allowing only five minutes of toilet time to become a conditioned reflex.

All in all, changing dietary habits and patterns is the best way to enable the process of elimination to function properly. Olive oil, commonly used in salad dressings, sauces, or to lightly sauté, is a natural diuretic containing little cholesterol. Chicory coffee is another natural diuretic and caffeine substitute. Other herbs which are digestive aids include basil (a staple of salads and Italian sauces) and elderberry and lovage, both great-tasting teas. Senna and pennyroyal may also do the trick but should be taken with care—and never if you are pregnant—since contractions and abdominal pain can result from excessive use. Although they may fulfill their promise, over-the-counter laxatives should be avoided as they can become addictive and, in high doses, may cause chronic diarrhea and severe stomach pains. Those designated as natural, or vegetable based, are safer since they are, in actuality, concentrated fiber. If you are a hemorrhoid sufferer, the following suggestions can be helpful in addition to dietary changes and glycerine suppositories.

1. A dab of petroleum jelly inserted approximately a half-inch using a Q-Tip acts as a lubricant to help the stool pass smoothly.
2. Cleanliness and good bowel habits are vital. Use soft white toilet tissue free of perfume. A wad of cotton soaked in ice-cold witch hazel will alleviate the pain caused by hemorrhoids.
3. When excessive sitting is unavoidable, use a doughnut-shaped cushion, readily available in pharmacies and medical supply establishments, to relieve the pressure.
4. At the end of the day, take a warm sitz bath—sitting with knees raised in three or four inches of warm water. The tepid water is soothing and increases the flow of blood to the area, which helps shrink the swelling. Aromatherapy oils such as juniper and bergamot added to the water will make a bath even more appealing.[9]

Although this condition is more uncomfortable than serious, constipation can be a symptom of more serious abdominal and colon disturbances. If constipation persists more than two weeks and/or if blood is present in the stool, it would be wise to consult a professional.

HEALING HERBS

There are a variety of herbs that are helpful to soothe common Scorpio ailments. Ginseng, a stimulant, blood purifier, and supposed aphrodisiac, is an herb Scorpios can use to stabilize their emotions rather than soaring to immeasurable highs and, afterward, catapulting to devastating lows. Kelp, a wonderful source of iodine, is a seaweed that can help the thyroid, reproductive organs, and cleanses the system. Kelp can be obtained in tablet or powder form and can be sprinkled over salads.

Other foods that aid Scorpios' digestion and the process of elimination are onions, watercress, cauliflower, leeks, turnips, radishes, figs, and prunes. Herbs that stimulate these functions are black mustard, chamomile, anise, caraway, coriander, fennel, ginger, goldenseal, marjoram, mustard, nutmeg, parsley, rosemary, and sage.

CLEANSING THE COLON

Aside from sporadic trips to the bathroom and lack of fiber in the diet, constipation can also result from hormonal imbalances, an underactive thyroid gland, pregnancy, and, more commonly, irritable bowel syndrome (IBS). Also known as spastic colon, IBS occurs when spasms of the colon prevent intestinal contents from moving through the digestive tract.

If spastic colon is not nipped in the bud, it can result in colitis, an inflammation of the colon, or large intestine, which is responsible for extracting nutrients and water from food before elimination occurs. Other causes of colon malfunction and colitis include emotional stress, lack of dietary fiber, too much fatty food, insufficient intake of water, and not enough physical activity to exercise the colon.

Colonics, or colon therapy (also called colon hydrotherapy), is a method of cleansing the large intestine of impurities using colonic irrigation with purified water. Vitamins, herbs, helpful bacteria, or oxygen may be added to the mixture as well. Enemas are utilized for the same purpose though they are not as powerful as complete irrigation. Once a popular means to cure colds and fevers, enemas, whose usage was replaced by antibiotics, are having a resurgence, and offer quick relief to ward off infections and purify the system. A gentle flow of water provided by an enema can loosen waste and dislodge toxins which would otherwise be released into the bloodstream and distributed throughout the body. The colon therapist simultaneously massages the colon through the abdomen to assist in the breakup of accumulated materials. This should not be done on a regular basis as overuse can be harmful.

Potassium, which aids in water elimination and activates production of digestive enzymes, is found in strawberries, asparagus, cantaloupe, bananas, oranges, almonds, potatoes, sesame seeds, and tuna fish. If you use colonics, or fast on a regular basis as a means of detoxification, be sure to take potassium supplements to replace lost electrolytes.

Other ways to cleanse the colon include the ingestion of certain herbs or other substances, such as psyllium seed husks or flax seeds, which loosen and break up stagnated materials in the colon. Acupuncture has proven to be very effective in activating the colon. A friend of mine who has been a colitis sufferer for years is convinced that once acupuncture sessions were added to her treatment (which consisted of medication and dietary changes), the condition vastly improved. (It is important to note that acupuncture is not a substitute for medication in the treatment of colitis.)

Crohn's disease, a chronic and often debilitating disorder which affects the small and large intestine, also comes under the category of inflammatory bowel disease (IBD). Although there is no known cure for this ailment, which, along with colitis, often goes through long periods of remission, the above recommendations plus dietary changes and stress relief cannot hurt.

YOGA EXERCISES

Scorpios can greatly benefit from the Abdominal Lift, a yogic exercise which maintains the resilience of your abdominal muscle and provides relief from constipation. Since it strengthens and stimulates the stomach, small intestine, colon, liver, kidneys, gallbladder, and pancreas, this asana is also recommended to Virgos, Librans, and Sagittarians. Abdominal lifts can be practiced in either a sitting or standing position as follows.

ABDOMINAL LIFT (SITTING POSITION)

1. Sit cross-legged while contracting your abdominal muscles as much as possible.
2. After exhaling all the air out of your lungs, suck in your abdomen by lifting the abdomen inward and then upward. You should feel your pelvis tilting upward and forward.
3. Hold that position for a few minutes.

4. Inhale and relax before exhaling and beginning the exercise again.
5. Repeat five times.

ABDOMINAL LIFT (STANDING POSITION)

1. Stand with knees slightly bent, heels together, toes pointed outward, and hands resting on the thighs.
2. After exhaling deeply, continue to gently press your hands down on your thighs while lifting the abdomen inward and upward at the same time. Again, you should feel your pelvis tilting and your spine elongating.
3. Inhale and straighten to the upright position.
4. Relax and repeat five times.

CYSTITIS

Since Scorpio rules the lower part of the body, there is a proclivity toward cystitis, urinary tract infections, and weakness in the bladder, prostate, ovaries, or fallopian tubes. Women are especially prone to cystitis (short for interstitial cystitis), an often chronic bladder disorder which arises when bacteria, viruses, and fungi in the urine attach themselves to the bladder wall. If the coating of the bladder, which prevents foreign substances from entering, is worn down, the bladder may become inflamed and irritated, manifested in itching and burning sensations, especially during urination. Cystitis and urinary tract infections are both characterized by an urgent need to pass water, and feelings of pressure, pain, and tenderness around the bladder when urinating and during intercourse. In the case of women, symptoms become more intense at the peak of the menstrual cycle. As with many other illnesses, stress may exacerbate symptoms.

Other than prescribed drugs and antibiotics, which will rid the body of bacteria, there are many natural methods that may be utilized to aid cystitis, urinary tract infections, and bladder problems. Since fluids top the list to fight the stinging sensation, it is advisable to drink six to eight glasses of water daily. Reduce the intake of foods with high acidic content such as alcohol, tomatoes, spices, chocolate, and caffeinated and citrus beverages, since they may contribute to bladder irritation and inflammation. Cranberry juice has been recommended to fight urinary tract infection primarily because it changes the urine's acidic content. In actuality, one would have to drink a voluminous amount in order for it to have any real effect. (However, it cannot hurt to add pleasant-tasting, unsweetened cranberry juice to your diet.) In addition to supplements of vitamin B complex and vitamin E, vitamin C is highly recommended for averting and eliminating bladder infections. Rose hips tea promotes healthy functioning of the bladder and kidneys. One of the best sources of ascorbic acid, rose hips also contain vitamins A, E, B_1, B_2, B_3, K, P, calcium, phosphorus, and iron.

Herbs like echinacea and golden seal are suggested for their ability to strengthen the immune system and help fight infection. Marshmallow root tea relieves inflammation of the urinary tract lining as do alfalfa, juniper, yarrow, and parsley. One cup of yogurt containing lactobacillus acidophilus, the live bacteria which functions as a natural antibiotic and fortifies the intestines and bladder, should be eaten daily. Be sure to check the label for this ingredient as it is not always added to yogurt sold in grocery stores or supermarkets. Yogurt sold in health food stores will almost always contain acidophilus. Because it contains vitamins A, B, D, and protein, yogurt with acidophilus may also aid in the treatment of constipation, kidney disorders, gallstones, and skin ailments.

If you live in a damp, windy climate and must be outdoors a great deal, dress warmly since exposure to chills may cause discomfort to the lower portion of the body. If you are caught in the rain, remove wet clothing the moment you get indoors and soak in a warm bath. Many cystitis sufferers claim that a regular exercise regime relieved their symptoms and, in some cases, hastened remission.

Since Scorpio rules the reproductive system, females may be prone to an irregular menstrual cycle, endometriosis, chlamydia, and general yeast infections; if you are male, prostitis or testicular complaints may be a problem. Since prostate cancer is the most common cancer in men, the American Cancer Society recommends that all men over the age of fifty have an annual checkup which involves a blood test to see if there is an elevation in the levels of PSA, a protein secreted by the prostate. African-American men and those with a family history should start the screening process at age forty to forty-five.

Women of childbearing age may be genetically predisposed to endometriosis, a reproductive system malfunction in which tiny pieces of the endometrium (uterine lining) escape from the uterus to the fallopian tubes, often leading to infertility if not timely or properly treated. Symptoms include cramping during periods and painful intercourse. Hormonal therapy, the main course of treatment, usually stops the progression of endometriosis and prevents infertility. Because this condition may worsen over time, women with endometriosis are usually advised not to delay having children too long if they wish to become parents.

MENOPAUSAL DISCOMFORT

Although menopause may be particularly stressful for many women, Scorpio females may be especially uncomfortable when production of estrogen and progesterone, the female hormones responsible for menstruation and ovulation, slows up and then stops. While menopause may occur between the ages of forty-five to fifty-five, symptoms can begin as early as age thirty-five, a period now labeled perimenopause. Loss of the hormonal cycle may range from psychological reactions like moodiness, depression, memory loss, and insomnia to physical changes like hot flashes, night sweats, and cramps. Once the menstrual cycle has completely stopped, you will experience thinning of hair, dry skin, loss of bone density, and general signs of aging. In addition to hormonal replacement therapy (see Chapter 11) and psychological counseling, there are many herbs which not only relieve depression and insomnia but contain phytoestrogens (natural plant estrogens) which actually mirror the effects of the missing hormones—but to a lesser extent. These herbs, which include black cohosh, licorice, and alfalfa, are completely safe.

In recent years, wild yam, which replicates the effects of progesterone, has been endorsed by many women going through perimenopause and menopause. Available in ointment form, this herb when rubbed on the belly has saved many women I know from the throes of mood swings and outright depression. It is also available in capsule or oil form. Of course, any remedies already mentioned in this book that relieve fatigue, depression, insomnia, and moodiness can be used to alleviate menopausal symptoms. Strenuous aerobic exercise is also recommended to Scorpios for tension relief and to stimulate endorphin production, which helps decrease moodiness, insomnia, and hot flashes.

AROMATHERAPY AND ESSENTIAL OILS

Since Scorpios are somber and intense, strong, sweet-smelling essential oils like orange blossom, rose, and jasmine can ease moodiness and depression when inhaled or added to the bathwater. Also called neroli, orange blossom is extracted via steam distillation from flowers of the orange blossom tree, which originated in China but now grows in France, California, and Italy. Neroli is also used as massage oil or to enliven tired skin. Rubbing it on the abdomen is said to relieve spasms.

Rose is one of the most expensive and magnificently fragrant essential oils. Without any awareness that the oil of a rose contains healing properties, many people instinctively place its petals in a dish of water so its magnificent aroma can permeate the room. Placing rose petals in water, inhaling rose oil, or utilizing its fragrance in the form of candles, incense, or potpourri is especially recommended for asthma sufferers. Massaging the chest, neck, and face with rose oil can elevate Scorpio moods and avert depression. If you suffer from insomnia, place a few drops on your pillow or dab a little under your nose before bedtime. Rubbing rose oil on your abdomen and lower back daily has been recommended to regulate the menstrual cycle.

Distilled from the Indian tree of the same name, sandalwood is a familiar incense scent. When sandalwood oil is inhaled and/or massaged on the stomach, throat, and chest, it eases nausea, vomiting, and coughing. Adding it to a hot bath can reduce stress, allowing you to sleep through the night. For relief from cystitis, constipation, and other aches, try rubbing juniper oil on the lower abdomen, or add five to six drops to the bathwater, making sure to soak in it for at least fifteen minutes. Bergamot bath oil may ease cystitis discomfort. For constipation, massage a blend of marjoram and lemon oil on the abdomen.

AYURVEDA

Most Scorpios can easily be classified as a combination of two Ayurvedic doshas—Pitta and Vata. Your hard-driven, ambitious side highlights the Pitta personality. Since Mars is the coruler of Scorpio, you, like most Pitta types, are characterized by high intensity and relentless physical energy. You thrive on challenges and often confront problems aggressively, which can undermine your productivity. When you are under a great deal of stress, you become more tense, and display a tendency toward fear and anger—emotions which are alternately repressed and released.

As a Vata type, you are sensitive to the environment but must maintain complete control, which, according to Ayurvedic philosophy, directly affects the bowels' inability to relax and function properly.

While your workaholism and constant need for activity can be productive and admirable, you will suffer from digestive complaints if your actions are motivated by anger or compulsion. Take a few minutes to unwind by meditating, breathing deeply, or simply closing your eyes and visualizing a remote, quiet beach. Cool yourself off by applying cool compresses on your forehead or on the back of your neck.

Because you are a combination of Pitta and Vata, you are encouraged to add sweet, Kapha-producing foods to your diet. According to Ayurveda, sweet foods include milk, cream, butter, whole-wheat bread, rice, honey, "sweet" vegetables (tomato, eggplant, sweet potato), and oil. This does not mean that you should eat an abundance of food high in fat and cholesterol. Try adding a bit of honey or butter to your foods, eating rice pudding, and having wheat bread and butter for breakfast. These simple dietary changes will slow you down and convert your anger to "sweeter" emotions. (For more information on Pitta and Vata types, see Chapters 2 and 4 on Aries and Gemini. After reading both descriptions, you can judge for yourself if you gravitate to one dosha more than the other.)

MINERAL SALT

The mineral salt for Scorpio is sulphate of lime (Calc. Sulph.). Also called calcium sulfate, this mineral salt, contained in the skin, mucous membranes, and tissue, purifies the body of toxins by helping the elimination process. Deficiencies may result in constipation, acne, and poor healing of bruises, cuts, and burns. Foods which contain calcium sulfate include onions, mustard, garlic, cauliflower, leeks, turnips, radishes, watercress, figs, kale, and prunes.

GEM AND COLOR THERAPY

If you were born between October 23 and October 31, your birthstone is the white opal, a translucent precious stone. If you were born between November 1 and November 22, your birthstone is the precious topaz, a yellow-brown semiprecious stone. Other gems associated with Scorpio are bloodstone, lodestone, malachite, jasper, and vermilion. The metal is plutonium. The color associated with Scorpio is black and represents the sign's melancholic, intense, and introverted side. Light-colored stones like opal and topaz, however, can elevate your moods and provide the optimism which often eludes you.

Chapter 10

Sagittarius the Archer

Aim for the Stars
but Don't Forget Your Body

SAGITTARIUS THE ARCHER
(NOVEMBER 23–DECEMBER 20)
RULING PLANET: Jupiter
ELEMENT: Fire
MODALITY: Mutable

Positive Sagittarius traits and concepts: forthright, optimistic, athletic, freedom-loving, intellectual, worldly, love of knowledge, teacher, philosophical, idealistic, generous, and hospitable.

Negative Sagittarius traits and concepts: insensitive, cavalier, abrasive, arrogant, know-it-all, fanatic, indulgent, messiah complex, dictatorial, excessive, irresponsible, and unrealistic.

Parts of the body ruled by Sagittarius include the hips, hamstrings, thighs, pelvis, liver, gallbladder, and sciatic nerve. Its ruling planet, Jupiter, governs the pituitary gland and the liver.

Ailments include obesity (especially around the hips), lower back problems, fractured hip, gallstones, alcoholism, and liver ailments, including cirrhosis, hepatitis, and jaundice.

Professions which appeal to Sagittarius' love of travel, learning, teaching, religion, and writing include teacher, professor, publisher, editor, journalist, writer, actor, director, motivational speaker, professional athlete, lawyer, evangelist, priest, and travel agent.

SAGITTARIUS THE ARCHER:
STAYING HAPPY THROUGH ETERNAL OPTIMISM

A mutable fire sign, Sagittarius the Archer is optimistic and open-minded yet excessive and fanatic about principles, beliefs, and anything about which he or she is passionate. Symbolized by the centaur—half-man, half-horse—which shoots idealistic arrows into the air, Sagittarians always aim upward and onward. Your altruism, sense of justice, inquisitiveness, and intelligence lead you to great conquests and enterprises. Wearing your ideals on your sleeve, you strive to change the world, but impracticality and restlessness often prevent you from implementing your goals in a pragmatic, meaningful way. Like the archer aiming his bow, this sign, both conformist and irreverent rebel, is always on the lookout for another mountain to climb and more knowledge to absorb. Freedom-loving, athletic, and philosophical, you will go to almost any length, and travel almost any distance, to pursue excitement, meet new people, and access information.

Whether involved in publishing, law, the performing arts, or education, Sagittarians, like yourself, are passionate about sharing what they've learned, relating travel anecdotes, or imparting spiritual lessons. A serious, informative teacher and an entertainer at heart, you easily captivate an audience with your wit, eloquence, and charm. Unfortunately, you often become didactic and preachy, offering unsolicited advice you think others should hear.

You are honest to a fault—even brutal—saying what is on your mind and/or correcting others' mistakes. At times, you are even fanatical and intolerant of differing points of view. Like your ruler, Jupiter, the Greco-Roman king of the gods, you often act as a law unto yourself, going so far as to make your own rules. You dislike being restricted, controlled, or limited. Believing you can conquer the world may be a wonderful confidence-building tool, but you must maintain humility and objectivity about yourself to avoid becoming megalomaniacal or fanatic. Although you are often opinionated and self-righteous, you are passionate in your beliefs and can motivate others to seek answers to their problems.

Whether you take academic courses, attain multiple degrees, or attend the school of hard knocks, you become bored unless you can learn and grow from every situation. Your quest for knowledge is so overwhelming that even your personal and professional relationships mirror the student/teacher relationship. Once you feel there is nothing more to learn or gain, your interest in the partnership ultimately wanes. Because of a never-ending need to impress and be impressed by others, you often appear to be a bon vivant and social climber, choosing friends and connections who you deem to be important, even powerful.

Like Aries and Leo, the other fire signs, you are exciting, passionate, romantic, and completely self-absorbed. Your personality, however, is comprised of two distinctly different facets. At a moment's notice, the flamboyance, magnanimity, and happy-go-lucky outlook can dissipate, and you become overly serious, judgmental, and dictatorial.

PHYSIOGNOMY AND BODY TYPE

Aristocratic and refined, the Sagittarian face has arched eyebrows, almond-shaped eyes, long nose, well-formed mouth, and pointed chin. You are usually medium to tall in height, and not particularly heavy, but Sagittarius rulership of the hips and thighs almost guarantees an hourglass, or pear-shaped, figure. Despite dieting and exercise, excess weight will immediately travel to the lower regions of the body, reaffirming that old adage "a moment on the lips, a lifetime on the hips." Pear-shaped figures, according to most experts, are not prone to heart or lung diseases, but have a tendency toward ailments affecting the kidneys, liver, pancreas, and reproductive organs—all of which comprise the lower section of the body. Since Sagittarius rules the thighs, hips, gallbladder, and liver, you may be forced to deal with overindulgence your entire life, and, as a result, be plagued by obesity, gallstones, diabetes, and liver disease—ailments caused or exacerbated by excess.

While you may search the world for spiritual teachings, you are also a thrill seeker who will mountain climb, join hiking expeditions, and go cross-country skiing in order to find excitement. As careful as you are about keeping your body in perfect shape to ensure stamina, you can be equally indulgent and remiss in taking care of yourself. With Jupiter, the planet representing abundance and appetite, as your ruler, you simply don't know when to stop eating, drinking, spending, or even gambling. Luckily, your thirst for adventure and need for excitement dictates that you remain supple and flexible.

LEARNING MODERATION

Since some of your problems stem from indulgence, it is very important to cut down on alcohol and fried foods, which can damage the Sagittarius-ruled liver and gallbladder. Tips for a balanced diet include reducing your intake of meat, dairy products, sugar, and salt; eating plenty of vegetables, fruits, and grain products. Try experimenting with a variety of satisfying recipes so you will not feel bored or deprived.

With all the entertaining, traveling, and dining out that Sagittarians do, it would be highly impractical to advise you to completely eliminate everything "interesting" from your diet. The key to healthily surviving cocktail parties, business luncheons, and dinners out is moderation—pure and simple. The following guidelines may help you to socialize without feeling robbed.

When you go out to dinner or attend a social function, cut the alcohol intake in half. An even better idea is switching to a nonalcoholic drink like tomato juice (with spices and lime), mineral water with lime, or diet cola with lemon. If you must have one glass of wine, drink spritzers, which are part carbonated water and part white wine. Pass up the high-calorie hors d'oeuvres at cocktail parties in favor of crudites—freshly cut vegetables which usually surround a tasty dip. Since the dip is usually loaded with calories and fat, use it sparingly.

When ordering in restaurants, take note of those dishes which appear to be low in calories but are secretly loaded with fat and sugar. Try not to select food cooked in a sauce since most sauces are comprised of sweeteners and thickening ingredients such as flour or cornstarch. Order poultry or fish that is broiled or grilled rather than fried or baked. Remove all visible skin from poultry. If you order broiled fish or meat, ask that it be cooked dry, with butter or sauce served on the side. When you order salad, the best dressing is oil and vinegar—also on the side.

While it may be embarrassing at first, it will soon become second nature to ask the server how a dish is prepared. Most of the time, he or she will provide the information willingly. It is more than likely that other diners are asking the very same questions. When you learn to practice moderation, you may be able to "cheat" every once in a while, as long as you get back on track immediately. Always remember that "excess" is your middle name.

TRAVEL TIPS

If you travel to exotic places with questionable sanitary conditions, refrain from drinking the water or eating fresh fruits and vegetables unless they are thoroughly washed and cooked in boiled water. Even bottled fruit juices are not a good idea. Instead, carry bottled water with you at all times, and be certain that everything you eat and drink has been boiled thoroughly. Sharing utensils will put you at risk of contracting infectious hepatitis (hepatitis A), which is not only incapacitating for anywhere from a few weeks to a few months but can cause irreversible liver damage and relapses for many years to come.

MAINTAINING A HEALTHY LIVER

Like Taurus, Cancer, Libra, and Pisces, the other indulgent signs, those born under Sagittarius often struggle a lifetime to control excessive habits, including too much food and alcohol, which can take the edge off life's stresses.

While you may not actually be afflicted with alcoholism, a physical and psychological ailment, you still may be drinking too heavily. If you find that you cannot get through the day without having a drink, or that you are convinced you can abstain at any time but prefer not to, you might seek counseling or the support of a group like Alcoholics Anonymous immediately before the situation worsens and your personal life suffers. (See Chapter 13 for more information on alcoholism.)

Serious ailments like hepatitis and cirrhosis of the liver (a deadly ailment resulting from extended alcohol abuse) may irreparably damage the liver, one of the most important organs in the body. If alcoholism continues over many years, liver cells die and are replaced with scar tissue, resulting in irreparable liver damage and, in the extreme, cirrhosis.

If you have diminished liver function, or vitamin deficiencies caused by excessive drinking, turn to protein and vitamin B, which act to regenerate the tissue and strengthen a fragile and substantially weakened nervous system. Vitamin C, potassium, and iron supplements will help anemia, which is often a byproduct of alcoholism.

HEALING HERBS

Milk thistle and turmeric have proven to be very effective in the liver's healing process. Used in European folk medicine for liver ailments, milk thistle and its extracts are still used to treat hepatitis and cirrhosis. Turmeric, a very hot spice used in Indian curries, contains the active ingredient curcumin, which researchers think may actually protect the liver by increasing the secretion of bile.

Chicory is a great noncaffeinated coffee substitute and a popular beverage in New Orleans. Utilized as a diuretic and laxative, its healing capacities extend to strengthening the liver and alleviating the aches and pains caused by gout and rheumatism. Additionally, chicory is reputed to dissolve gallstones and eliminate excess mucus. Bay leaves, which are absolutely essential for casseroles and stews, are thought to stimulate the spleen and the liver, while their oil can be used to heal bruises.

A blood purifier, mild laxative, and digestive aid, the root and leaves of the dandelion have been used by herbalists throughout the world to treat liver, gallbladder, and spleen dysfunction. Literally meaning lion's tooth (from the French *dent de lion*), the dandelion, which blossoms in late spring, is native to Europe and Asia but has been cultivated throughout the world to become one of the most recognizable flowers. The medicinal properties of the dandelion root and its leaves were originally recorded in medical journals by Arab physicians in the tenth century. During the sixteenth century, British herbalists considered the plant a valuable diuretic, and by the nineteenth century dandelion became recognized both in Europe and in America.

Fluids extracted from dandelion root are used to make juice and wine. The roots can be cleaned, dried, roasted, ground, and substituted for coffee or as an ingredient in hot chocolate. Dandelion leaves can be steeped as tea, added to salads, steamed, or sautéed. They are rich in calcium, phosphorus, iron, potassium, and vitamins A, B, and C. Dandelion can treat obesity, gout, hypertension, arteriosclerosis, and kidney stones. The leaves are also used for facials and in herbal baths.

GALLSTONES

With Sagittarius ruling the liver and gallbladder, you are a perfect candidate for gallstones. Composed of bile (secreted by the liver to help break down fats for digestion) and cholesterol or calcium deposits in the liver or gallbladder, gallstones can be as tiny as a grain of sand or as large as an egg. Most of the time stones pass through the system unnoticed. Pain is produced when they become lodged in the passages which connect the gallbladder with the liver, pancreas, and intestine. The obstruction will induce an attack without warning, resulting in inflammation, nausea, vomiting, and severe right-upper-abdominal pain often radiating to the right shoulder or back. Most susceptible to gallstones are those who are overweight, have diabetes, or women who've had children—though I know people who do not fall into any of these categories but have nonetheless been afflicted.

An attack can occur between fifteen to sixty minutes after eating, especially if the food is fatty or fried. Sufferers should avoid large meals high in fat, which aggravate this condition. The diet should be high in protein, carbohydrates, and fluids, preferably six to eight glasses of water daily. Fat soluble vitamins A, D, E, and K are recommended since they assist in absorbing fats. Vitamin A is readily obtainable in carrots, spinach, and broccoli; vitamin D can be found in milk and fish liver oil; vitamin E is contained in seeds, nuts, soybeans, and vegetable oils; and vitamin K is found in most leafy green vegetables, milk, yogurt, and egg yolks. Needless to say, you can also take vitamin supplements.

LECITHIN

A phospholipid comprised of saturated, unsaturated, and polyunsaturated fatty acids, lecithin produces linoleic acid, the essential fatty acid the body requires to metabolize cholesterol, triglycerides, and other lipids, thereby preventing the formation of gallstones, arterial plaque buildup, and atherosclerosis (See Chapter 6.). Often called "brain food," lecithin is a nutrient high in phosphorus. When combined with iron, iodine, and calcium, it invigorates the brain, aids digestion, increases immunity against viral infections, and transports nutrients from the bloodstream into cells. Lecithin is found naturally in the myelin sheath, the fatty protective covering of the nerves, and is thought to play an important part in the maintenance of a healthy nervous system.

With an ability to cleanse the liver and purify the kidneys, lecithin is contained in egg yolk, soybeans, corn, cabbage, calves' liver, cauliflower, caviar, eggs, garbanzo beans (chickpeas), green beans, lentils, rice, and split peas and can be taken as a supplement in capsule, liquid, and granule forms. Because gallstones are aggravated by high levels of fat, it is beneficial to obtain lecithin from vegetables, grains, and beans rather than from animal products.

Parsley, a well-known herb used in cooking and salads, is an excellent diuretic and valuable in the treatment of gallbladder problems. Available in leaves, roots, and seeds, this condiment is usually added to salads, sauces, and casseroles.

GOUT

Because Jupiter rules expansion, there is a tendency for Sagittarians to develop a variety of growths, warts, cysts, tumors, and gout—a form of arthritis where the joint becomes swollen, tender, and excruciatingly painful. Gout arises from excess uric acid, which crystallizes and inflames the joints, causing swelling, throbbing, and excruciating pain. While gout can afflict anyone, it is most common among overweight, middle-aged men. It is important to note that any condition which may be aggravated or caused by excess pounds comes under the auspices of Sagittarius.

The most immediate preventive measure is to reduce the levels of uric acid by eliminating food containing purine, the substance in which the acid is contained. Foods high in purine include high-protein animal products such as anchovies, brains, consommé, gravy, heart, herring, kidney, liver, meat extracts, mussels, mincemeat, sardines, and sweetbreads.

If you suffer from gout or any other swelling, apply an ice pack, elevate your leg, and take a simple anti-inflammatory like ibuprofen. If your stomach reacts adversely to it, refrain from using it immediately. Soaking your foot in warm water with charcoal added is therapeutic, as is the application of charcoal poultices, which are said to draw toxins from the body. Drinking plenty of fluids and herbal teas such as sarsaparilla, yarrow, rose hip, and peppermint is also recommended for relieving the inflammation.

RELIEVE SCIATICA AND LOWER BACK PAIN

Sciatica refers to severely painful spasms along the sciatic nerve, which extends from the back of the thigh down the inside of the leg to the ankle. Causes of sciatica are trauma or inflammation of the nerve, sprained joints in the lower back, and rupture of a disk between the spinal bones, or neuritis. Pain caused by injury to the lower back or from a slipped disk is much more intense if pressure is being placed on the sciatic nerve.

Treatment for sciatica includes rest, the application of ice packs to the affected leg for relief of pain and inflammation; and vitamin B complex to strengthen the nerves. (See Chapter 6 for tips on healing a slipped disk.)

Yoga Asanas

Since it is the perfect tool for purifying mind and body, yoga appeals to the Sagittarian ideal of attaining both physical and spiritual perfection. Sagittarius rules the thighs, hips, hamstrings, and sciatic nerve; yoga positions and exercises which strengthen these areas will not only lessen the pain in the legs caused by sciatica, but also in the lower back since the nerves are being stretched simultaneously. The following yoga asanas are a few of the many positions which are utilized for strengthening those parts of the body and which can ease the excruciating pain that sciatica often inflicts.

The Bow (Dhanurasana) (Fig 10.1)

The Bow, or Dhanurasana (literally meaning "Archer posture"), in which the body is pulled tautly like a bowstring, stretches and strengthens the inner thighs and hamstrings. For Sagittarians, who are plagued by problems relating to thighs, hamstrings, and the sciatic nerve, the following position is tailor-made.

1. Lie flat on your abdomen and chest with chin on the floor and knees spread apart.
2. Flex the legs and bring the heels back close to the buttocks.
3. Grasp your ankles firmly, with thumbs and fingers side by side.

4. Lift head, neck, and shoulders as high as you can, and at the same time pull firmly on ankles.
5. Keep your arms straight and lift thighs and chest clear off the floor to balance on your stomach.
6. Hold yourself in this drawn-bow position for at least six seconds.

If practiced regularly, Dhanurasana will increase circulation and elongate the hip joints, back, thighs, shoulders, and spine. In addition, the front of the body, including the legs, abdomen, throat, and pelvic area, are stretched.

THE HEADSTAND

Urdhva Dandasana (the "Raised Spine" pose), a headstand in which the legs are extended at a 90-degree angle to the body rather than overhead, is a fabulous asana for stretching the spine and for working the thighs and hamstrings.

1. Set a mat up against the wall.
2. Kneel on the mat with your back toward the wall. Leave enough room for your legs to be extended out from the wall.
3. Place the crown of your head on the mat.
4. Clasp your hands around your head directly beneath your hips and position your body as if you were about to do a headstand.
5. Slowly walk your feet up the wall until you form a right angle between your legs and your torso.
6. Press the soles of your feet against the wall.
7. Keep breathing and hold this position for about ten minutes, or less if it is uncomfortable.

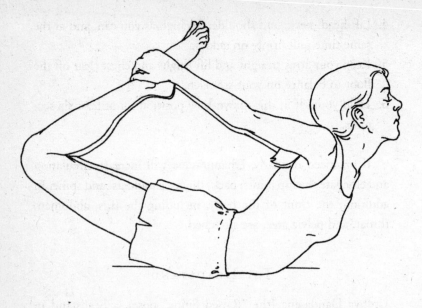

FIGURE 10.1 THE BOW (DHANURASANA)

If you are a beginner, it is important that your feet rest against a wall. If you are a yoga adept or an exercise aficionado, you may not need the wall. Do not attempt this exercise if you have high blood pressure or problems with your back, neck, or shoulders.

Lower back problems may also stem from tight hamstrings, which pull on the lower back. As the leg muscles lose elasticity and strength, they leave you vulnerable to knee and hip injuries. Fortunately, many problems can be avoided with regular practice of the following exercise which stretches the hamstrings.

The Ham Stretch, as it is called, can be done anywhere using a chair, table, and even the stairs. Because the hamstrings are inflexible, this exercise should be done more than once a day. It can even be practiced while performing other activities like talking on the phone.

1. Stand about two feet behind a chair with the seat facing you.
2. With your weight balanced, straighten your left foot on the seat, extend it through the heel.
3. If you do not feel a stretching sensation up the back of your left leg, rest your hands on your leg and lean forward at the hips until you feel the stretch. Hold the stretch while you inhale and exhale twice.
4. Remove your leg from the chair, relax it, and then repeat the stretch with the right leg.

AROMATHERAPY AND ESSENTIAL OILS

Used for years as a household disinfectant, juniper oil can also be utilized to stimulate circulation and relieve the troubling symptoms of gout and liver disorders. It works best when added to the bath and, in the case of gout, to any solution in which you may be soaking your feet. Juniper is also recommended for eradicating cellulite, pockets of unwanted fat which appear on your thighs and buttocks. Massage a blend of juniper, fennel, and lemon oil onto these areas after a bath when the skin is warm and sensitive. Fennel can be used as both an essential oil, as a condiment in stews and salads, or eaten as an after-dinner digestive aid. Sage, red clover, and jasmine oil also work well for Sagittarians.

AYURVEDA

According to Ayurvedic principles, Sagittarians may be classified as a combination of Kapha and Pitta doshas. Jupiter, the ruler of Sagittarius, is a jovial yet overindulgent planet, which fits the Kapha profile. As a dynamic fire sign, Sagittarius also fits the Pitta profile, which is enterprising and forthright. Since Sagittarius spans these two categories, the application of good living habits according to Ayurvedic principles can be attained by balancing both Kapha and Pitta doshas, though you probably lean more to the Kapha personality.

Although you are ambitious and enterprising, you are less hotheaded and aggressive than pure Pitta types. As long as you get enough exercise and fresh air to offset your natural laziness, you will be steady, purposeful, and will have the ability to accomplish your goals. Naturally relaxed, you suffer from the slings and arrows of constant procrastination and a tendency toward lethargy. If you suffer from water retention, exhaustion, fevers, and/or colds (a combination of Kapha and Pitta ailments), introduce astringent and bitter foods into the diet to increase Vata and decrease Kapha and Pitta. (See Appendix II.)

Eat more bitter foods, which stimulate digestion and counteract water retention, including endive, romaine lettuce, spinach, tonic water, and spices like turmeric and fenugreek. In place of caffeine, try chicory coffee and ginger tea. Astringent foods, which stimulate the colon, include beans, lentils, cabbage, broccoli, cauliflower, potatoes, apples, and pears. (See Chapters 3 and 4 on Aries and Taurus for more information on Pitta and Kapha types. After reading the descriptions, you can see which dosha may be more dominant in your personality.)

MINERAL SALT

Naturally found in the hair, nails, and skin, the Sagittarius mineral salt is silicic oxide (silica), important for maintaining the covering of bones and nerves. Boils, sties, brittle nails, and lifeless hair are signs of either a silica deficiency or that the salt is not being assimilated properly. Silica can be obtained from asparagus, parsnips, cucumbers, onions, whole wheat, strawberries, barley, rye, red cabbage, cherries, bran, and fruit and vegetable skins.

GEM AND COLOR THERAPY

If you are born between November 23 and November 30, your birthstone is the topaz, a yellow-gold semiprecious stone. If you were born between December 1 and 20, your birthstone is the turquoise, a bluish semiprecious stone mined throughout the Southwest, which, with coral and silver, are the main components of Native American jewelry. Jupiter, the ruler of Sagittarius, is associated with yellow and gold. Other stones with a yellowish hue which can be worn to heal Jupiterian ailments include amber, citrine, and yellow sapphire—an exquisite, precious gem. Although jaundiced skin, a symptom of a malfunctioning, Sagittarian-ruled liver, has a yellow cast, this very same color, obtained by wearing gems or bathing under a yellow light, is nonetheless used to provide energy to that organ. If you do wish to use gems, set these particular stones in gold and be certain that the gem is touching the skin. Not only will these Jupiterian stones invigorate the production of bile (which, in turn, stimulates digestion) but they will provide the eternal optimism which pervades the Sagittarian philosophy of life.

Chapter 11

Capricorn the Goat

The Ambitious Mountain Climber
with Brittle Bones

♑

CAPRICORN THE MOUNTAIN GOAT
(DECEMBER 21–JANUARY 19)
RULING PLANET: Saturn
ELEMENT: Earth
MODALITY: Cardinal

Positive Capricorn traits and concepts are ambitious, persevering, steady, stable, consistent, reserved, conservative, sensual, practical, work-oriented, disciplined, frugal, and goal-oriented.

Negative Capricorn traits and concepts are ruthless, workaholic, cold, arrogant, pessimistic, depressive, stodgy, stingy, selfish, lonely, and uncommunicative.

Parts of the body ruled by Capricorn include the knees, bones, skin, gums, and teeth. Its ruling planet, Saturn, governs the entire skeletal system.

Ailments include arthritis, fibromyalgia, rheumatism, osteo-porosis, neuritis, neuralgia, lupus, knee trouble, gingivitis, and tooth and gum disease.

Professions which appeal to Capricorn's efficiency, practicality, and organizational skills include executive, businessperson, real estate developer, researcher, scientist, priest, writer, and work which involves solitude.

CAPRICORN THE GOAT: AMBITION HELPS YOU CLIMB THE LADDER OF SUCCESS

Symbolized by a goat slowly climbing the mountain of success, Capricorn, a cardinal earth sign, is ambitious, steady, and reliable, plotting every move judiciously and butting every obstacle until the goal is attained. With Saturn, the Greco-Roman god of time, as your ruling planet, you are extremely disciplined, serious, and possess an amazing work ethic and sense of morality. While these attributes work to your advantage when a job must be done, you can be a difficult task master.

Authoritarian, judgmental, and extremely stern, you place high, almost unrealistic expectations on yourself and others. A pessimistic attitude and conservative approach to life is not particularly beneficial since you can be too judgmental and severe in your treatment of others. Your fastidiousness demands that you work painstakingly slow, and no matter how hard you try, or how diligent you work, time is elusive and always catches you in its trap.

Because of your cool exterior, reticence, and reserved personality, you are often regarded as aloof, distant, even cold. Privately, however, you are passionate and sensual, attesting to Capricorn's categorization as a visceral, earth sign.

Unable to easily trust or spontaneously express yourself, you are prudent and selective in revealing your deepest emotions. Once a friend or lover wins your confidence, you are completely at ease, open and affectionate—a far cry from the image presented to the outside world. You are a sincere and loyal friend, and your relationships span many years—sometimes as far back as childhood.

Loving and devoted, you always give your partner the benefit of the doubt and will not admit defeat nor abandon a relationship until all alternatives have been explored. On the other hand, you will not tolerate or excuse disloyalty. You may forgive, but you will certainly never forget.

Lacking spontaneity, you tend to withhold opinions until you have weighed each situation very carefully. Capricorns never fully divulge their feelings and speak only when they have something worthwhile to say. In fact, work is so overridingly important that emotions always take second place. Certainly a professional plus, this attitude takes its toll on your personal life. Too often work responsibilities take precedence over relationships.

A creature of habit and routine, you are adverse to change and are extremely uncompromising when it comes to new ideas, patterns, or even trying new food. This inflexibility can be harmful since your bones are as rigid as your personality. A tendency to worry about money, your job, and just about everything under the Sun is responsible for the frown lines on your face and for certain funks and periods of depression, which become overwhelming from time to time. Mental depression and feelings of hopelessness can be as debilitating as physical illness. Taking exercise, herbs, and relaxing and having fun will enhance your well-being. (See Chapter 7 for tips on depression.)

PHYSIOGNOMY AND BODY TYPE

You are usually medium in height and, more often than not, wiry with a bony structure. With Saturn-ruled Capricorn reigning over the skeletal system, joints, gums, teeth, skin, and knees, cheekbones are high and pronounced. You have deep-set eyes, a pug nose, and thin lips. Due to a conservative attitude toward life, you tend to dress casually, often selecting dark colors such as navy blue and black, avoiding bright hues and clothes which are ostentatious or low cut. In fact, your manner of dress directly reflects the desire to avoid attention. You prefer to stay behind the scenes pursuing your goals deliberately and single-mindedly. While you may not stand out in a crowd (due to your unassuming manner), your perseverance, ambition, and burning desire to achieve will eventually elevate you head and shoulders above the rest.

Conservative and moderate, you usually eat three balanced meals a day and exercise regularly. If under stress, you tend to undereat or skip meals altogether. Given your ambitions and the high standards you set for yourself, it is vital that you maintain the strength to endure the long hours which work frequently demands. Fatigue due to lack of proper nutrients could threaten your mental and physical health. If you are under pressure and happen to forget to eat, be certain to take protein supplements such as spirulina and bee pollen. Combining milk, eggs, and bananas in an electric blender and drinking the mixture will supply the calcium, potassium, and protein to replace the missing nutrients.

OSTEOPOROSIS

Your stiff character and stalwart personality often translate physically into bone and joint rigidity, especially later in life, when Capricorns are prone to diseases that affect the joints, bones, and skeletal system such as osteoarthritis, rheumatism, and, in the case of women, osteoporosis. Osteoporosis, a condition resulting from gradual bone loss, affects a large percentage of postmenopausal women, whose bones become brittle due to the negligible production of estrogen, a hormone that protects the skeletal system and the heart. This condition is further exacerbated by calcium deficiency, tobacco use, and lack of weight-bearing exercise, which helps increase bone density.

Once the process of bone loss begins, the skeletal system becomes fragile, inches are lost from the body, and the risk that you will lose your balance and fall, resulting in hip, spine, wrist, and other bone fractures, increases drastically.

Although all women are at risk, Capricorn women are especially susceptible since, as a rule, they are all "skin and bones," with fewer protective layers of fat. While 80 percent of osteoporosis sufferers are women, men over fifty are also vulnerable.

Since calcium is the most important mineral for strengthening the bones, a calcium-rich diet prior to the age of thirty-five may help prevent the onset of osteoporosis at a later age. Milk and milk products are loaded with calcium but are also high in fat and cholesterol. The good news is that low-fat cheese, yogurt, and milk offer the same amount of calcium as regular dairy products. Skim-milk products contain no fat at all, and you can even add powdered nonfat, dry milk to soups and sauces for additional calcium. Other sources that do not contain fat and cholesterol include salmon, sardines, nuts, tofu, oranges, broccoli, kale, spinach, and tomatoes. If you cannot get enough calcium from your diet alone, calcium carbonate tablets—an over-the-counter supplement—may work for you. The Recommended Dietary Allowance (RDA) for post-menopausal women is 1,200 to 1,400 milligrams.

Vitamin D, readily obtained in milk and sunlight, is necessary for the absorption of calcium. Magnesium and vitamin K also help to keep bones healthy. On the other hand, high levels of animal protein, sodium, refined sugar, and caffeine cause the elimination of calcium, and their intake should be reduced, if not deleted from the diet. Phosphorus also prevents calcium absorption, and foods high in this mineral such as meat, fish, eggs, poultry, seeds, and nuts should be reduced. Silica, an herb obtained in tea, homeopathic tinctures, or capsule form will help the body to absorb calcium as will alfalfa, black cohosh, wild yam, and comfrey.

In addition to increasing calcium intake, weight lifting under the supervision of a fitness professional at a gym or health club can increase bone density. If time constraints prevent you from joining a public facility, there are weight-lifting exercises which can be done at home using barbells, hand weights, or even tin cans. Additionally, there are a wide variety of instructional videos on the market which will guide you through these exercises. Yoga asanas are also invaluable as a means for increasing bone density and building stamina.

Other forms of exercise which strengthen bones include bike riding, running, swimming, even walking—the latter of which can be done almost effortlessly. Walking two miles per day—the equivalent of forty city blocks—can improve your overall health as well as fortify the skeletal system. Make extra time during the day to walk to activities instead of taking public transportation or an automobile. Use the stairs instead of an elevator or escalator whenever possible.

Hormone replacement therapy, which supplements the estrogen lost after menopause, can compensate but not completely substitute for loss of bone density, which must be attended to earlier in life through exercise and calcium intake. While estrogen replacement lubricates the skin, prevents heart disease, and thwarts bone loss, it may also increase the risk of certain types of breast cancer. If you feel you may benefit from estrogen replacement, study the pros and cons carefully by paying particular attention to the medical history of both you and your family. Before you decide to take this important step, it is an absolute must to do your own in-depth research and to consult your physician.

ARTHRITIS

One of the most painful and debilitating diseases to which Capricorns are prone is arthritis, an umbrella term that encompasses many disorders affecting the joints. Although this disease usually strikes as we get older, arthritis also afflicts a good portion of young adults. A chronic ailment with no known cause or cure, arthritis is an inflammation of one or more joints which produces a variety of symptoms from mild aches and stiffness to severe pain and crippling deformity.

Arthritis can be classified as either osteoarthritis or rheumatoid arthritis.

1. Osteoarthritis, a degenerative joint disease and the most common arthritic disorder, occurs when the cartilage between the bones deteriorates, permitting the bones to rub together when the joints are flexed, causing pain, swelling, and limited movement. It usually affects the fingers and joints of the knees, feet, hips, and back.

2. Rheumatoid arthritis, an autoimmune disease (when one part of the body attacks another part) where the inflammation of the joint lining causes deterioration of cartilage and bone, is the most debilitating form of this disease. Like osteoarthritis, the resulting joint pain can be excruciating, targeting the hands, wrists, feet, knees, ankles, shoulders, and elbows.

Although there is no actual cure for arthritis, traditional doctors usually prescribe powerful anti-inflammatory drugs to decrease joint swelling. While some of these drugs do alleviate the pain and swelling, the side effects may include nausea, stomach cramps, and general indigestion. Stress management and relaxation techniques like biofeedback, acupuncture, yoga, meditation, guided imagery, deep breathing, and even hypnotherapy strengthen the nervous system and alleviate stress. These methods all help to relax the tightened muscles around the joints so the sufferer can concentrate less on the pain. The degree of pain may actually diminish, improving the ability to cope. Relaxation can also assuage insomnia and depression—common symptoms of chronic pain sufferers. Biofeedback can help sufferers to recognize the onset of pain before its effects actually occur. Once the patient is alerted to the signals, relaxation techniques can then be applied.

Massage is a therapeutic means of relaxation which can be used to loosen the joints. If you cannot locate a professional, learn how to massage your fingers, elbows, and knees and to work the muscles that are attached to the tendons leading to your painful joints. Deep-tissue manipulation may be the perfect form of massage to energize and relax different parts of your body.

The National Institutes of Health's Office of Alternative Medicine has publicly endorsed acupuncture as a remedy for relieving the pain caused by arthritis. Acupuncture restores energy flow to affected joints. Studies have found that those who have undergone acupuncture treatments have far less discomfort than those who have not.

Research has also shown that a healthy, balanced diet may strengthen the immune system and, in the case of arthritis, limit inflammation. Because arthritis affects the joints, it is recommended that zucchini, tomatoes*, green peppers, eggplant, and white potatoes be eliminated from the diet due to their high acid content. Also called the nightshade vegetables, they are believed to deposit acid in the joints, exacerbating arthritis pain. Animal protein should also be cut out since it contains both arachidonic acid and phosphorus, which, as already stated, prevent calcium absorption. Calcium helps strengthen the bones, and supplements should be taken early in life if you are prone to this disease.

Since osteoarthritis inflicts enormous pain but has little to do with inflammation, Tylenol (generic acetaminophen) is the recommended over-the-counter painkiller rather than Advil (generic ibuprofen) which is an anti-inflammatory and recommended for rheumatoid arthritis. Since excess pounds cause more rapid deterioration of joints and cartilage, aerobic exercise and weight loss can help alleviate further inflammation, swelling, and arthritic pain. Exercise stimulates endorphin production, which makes one feel happier, and as a result pain is less intense. Stretching exercises and yoga asanas which target the affected joints are also beneficial. Other related conditions which may afflict Capricorns include fibromyalgia and gout (both forms of arthritis), rheumatism, tendinitis, pinched nerves, and lupus.

---

* Even though tomatoes contain calcium, they should be avoided due to high acidic content. There are many other foods as well as supplements which provide calcium.

HEALING HERBS

Herbs which may alleviate arthritic pain include willow bark and meadowsweet leaves, both of which contain natural salicylates. Sarsaparilla, a great-tasting tea, has also proved effective in relieving some of the symptoms of arthritis. Transported to the West Indies from Europe in the sixteenth century, this herb was first used as a cure for syphilis. It has since been found to relieve itching caused by skin inflammations like psoriasis, and recommended for inflammatory ailments such as gout, rheumatism, and arthritis. It is available in tablets, tincture, and as a flavorful extract which can be added to medicine and soft drinks. Used throughout the world, the most common varieties are grown in Jamaica, North America, and India. Cold compresses and massaging the joints with eucalyptus oil may help as well.

Ingestion of fish oil capsules has been known to decrease joint tenderness and fatigue in arthritis patients. Omega-3 fatty acids, the active ingredient in fish oil, is contained in cod liver oil and has been around for years. One teaspoon per day may help alleviate rheumatoid arthritis pain by providing substantial amounts of vitamin D—important for bone growth—and vitamin A, which may have anti-inflammatory effects. It is important to take the recommended dietary allowances of these vitamins since overages can cause liver damage. If you opt for cod liver oil, be prepared to place a cool mint in your mouth immediately after swallowing or else you will be left with an unpleasant aftertaste. Vitamin C may also stagnate the progression of rheumatoid arthritis.

Comfrey, also called boneset, is a plant indigenous to Europe and Asia which derives its nickname from the ability to strengthen cartilage and heal broken bones. High in protein, comfrey is used as a tea, dried herb and root, or in a cream or tincture. Applying comfrey oil or cream to the affected areas may help in the treatment of osteoporosis and arthritis.

Dandelion is a remarkable herb that can be utilized in many forms. Its leaves can be eaten in salads, and the juice, which is obtained from the leaves, is recommended to arthritis sufferers since it is said to break up acid deposits in the joints. Dandelion root is often roasted and ground to make a coffeelike drink which can also assuage arthritic pain.

Some theorists say that arthritic pain is exacerbated by a deficiency of copper, which sufferers cannot properly metabolize. Since they are unable to obtain the mineral from food, it is recommended by some that arthritis patients wear copper bracelets, by which the element enters the body to provide pain relief. While some professionals remain skeptical, most do not dismiss the theory entirely.

AROMATHERAPY AND ESSENTIAL OILS

It is of utmost importance that specific aromatherapy oils be used when you are getting or giving a massage. Juniper, thyme, hyssop, and chamomile oils are all recommended for the afflicted joints and the surrounding areas. For additional effectiveness, add a few drops of any of these oils to your bath.

Indigenous to France and Spain, rosemary is a popular cooking herb and salad flavoring as well as an essential oil distilled from the plant's flowers and leaves. It is not only a wonderful massage oil but a popular ingredient in shampoo and hair tonic, and is purported to improve scalp circulation and dandruff. To alleviate dandruff, massage the scalp with rosemary oil and leave it on for about thirty minutes before shampooing. When added to bathwater, it aids the circulation of the entire body.

Native to Central and South America, capsicum, the source

of cayenne pepper, has also been used in ointment form for osteoarthritis sufferers, who have actually attested to a reduction of joint pain. It is available as a tincture or in capsule form. The anti-inflammatory properties of feverfew make this herb, which grows wild in Europe and the United States, perfect for allaying arthritic pain. It is available as tincture, capsule, and tea.

Avoiding Knee Injuries

While you are quite athletic, and attracted to running and contact sports like football and soccer, be cautious of scrapes and injuries to the knees—a body part ruled by Capricorn. Your legs may be extremely strong, but your knees are particularly vulnerable and the first to go, especially if you already have arthritis or other joint sensitivities. If you partake in these sports, wear knee pads and soak your knees after each game or activity. Should you experience some of the warning signs that your arthritis is acting up, follow the dietary and herbal tips mentioned, and see your doctor immediately.

Gentle stretching exercises and yoga asanas are certain to make the joints more limber. The following simple exercise stretches the muscles around your knees and thighs:

1. Sit in an upright position with the soles of your feet touching.
2. Straighten your back and slowly pull your feet in toward you as far as you possibly can.
3. Lower your knees very slowly and gradually so that they are as close to the floor as they will go. Your thighs should start to feel tight. Push them down as far as you can without causing yourself undue pain.
4. Sit as erect as possible and hold this position for fifteen to twenty minutes or as long as possible.

5. Each time you try this exercise, you should be able to lower your knees a little farther. It is most important that you feel your knees and thighs stretching and extending where they do not normally go.

PERIODONTAL DISEASE

Capricorn's rulership of the skeletal system also extends to the teeth and the gums. Gingivitis, a condition characterized by bleeding, puffy, red gums, is the precursor to periodontal disease and, according to the American Dental Association, one of the main reasons adults lose their teeth. The primary cause of gingivitis is the buildup of plaque between the teeth and at the gumline due to improper brushing and insufficient flossing. Bacteria contained in plaque emit an acid which subsequently attacks tooth enamel, leading to thinner gums, tooth decay, and, at the extreme, loosening of the teeth. Sensitive, bleeding gums usually occur at a young age but can be prevented from becoming full-blown gingivitis if you adhere to the following simple guidelines.

1. To obtain the best results from brushing, use a small toothbrush with soft bristles which, when held at a 45-degree angle, will reach and clean teeth and gums simultaneously. Some experts advocate an electric toothbrush and contend that twice as much plaque can be removed electrically than by hand. While the electric toothbrush is a good preventive device, it may be too harsh and painful a tool for those already suffering from gingivitis.
2. Brush and floss after every meal. Scraping the tongue with a dull—never a sharp—instrument from back to front several times a day may also dislodge the germs which collect there.
3. Use the thumb and forefinger to massage and stimulate the

gums. Aromatherapy oils and herbs can also ease inflammations.

4. Reduce or completely eliminate alcohol and smoking, which
   deplete the body of vitamins and minerals essential to healthy
   teeth.

5. High doses of calcium strengthen the teeth and vitamin C
   fortifies the gums by preventing bleeding. In addition to citrus fruits like lemon, oranges, grapefruit, and tomatoes, the
   best source of vitamin C is rose hips, available in tea or capsules.

6. Rinsing with a store-bought mouthwash may reduce the
   buildup of plaque and help prevent gingivitis.

For those who already have this condition, the best advice is
to continue to brush and floss after each meal, and visit a dental
hygienist or periodontist four times per year. Increased bleeding,
a tooth which seems to have grown in size, receding gumlines, or
bad breath are signs that the gingivitis has worsened and professional help should be sought.

SKIN CONDITIONS

Unlike Librans, who often get acne and rashes due to excess
oils and toxins, Capricorn skin problems are usually due to
allergies, nervousness, and hypersensitivity. Because the skin becomes dry, chapped, and itchy in the winter, it is important for
Capricorns to use moisturizing cream or lotion on their hands,
feet, neck, and face. Common nonchemical lubricants such as
petroleum jelly, vitamin E oil, and aloe vera should be applied after bathing, before going outdoors, and prior to bed. Utilize sun-
block and sunscreen to prevent the skin from drying and protect
it from the harsh wind in winter and strong sun in summer.

Aloe vera is an herb that grows wild throughout Africa and the Mediterranean. It is best recognized as a moisturizing gel, ointment, or lotion which soothes itchy skin, rashes, blemishes, sunburn, burns, sores, and poison ivy. Used in Greece and presently grown throughout the Middle East, South America, southern Florida, and Texas, aloe vera stimulates epidermal growth and repairs dead skin cells. In addition to using preparations on the market, you can reward your skin with fresh gel by breaking off an aloe vera leaf and slicing it down the middle.

PSORIASIS

Often mistaken for severe dry skin, psoriasis is a persistent, non-contagious skin disorder characterized by a thick, scaly buildup of skin cells called plaques, which are red and often itchy. Most prevalent on the scalp, elbows, knees, and buttocks, psoriasis results when skin cells run amok and are "out of control." Normally, it takes about thirty days for a new skin cell to work its way from the lowest layer to the surface. In psoriasis, cells reach the top layer in three days. While they die like normal cells, they are so overabundant that the plaques become white and flaky as they fluff off. Psoriasis often goes through sequences of flare-ups and remissions, sometimes disappearing for months or years and either improving or worsening with age. Since stress can trigger the outbreak of psoriasis, tension-alleviating techniques mentioned throughout this book will help.

Due to the ailment's unknown cause, there is, at the present time, no permanent cure. There are, however, a variety of remedies which will relieve the itching and burning sensations. Available over the counter, a mixture of Indian earth and moisturizing lotion applied on the inflamed elbows and knees can provide relief and camouflage the unsightly plaques. The discomfort of itching and flaking can be relieved with emollients like baby oil, vegetable shortening, petroleum jelly, and vitamin E oil, which should be rubbed onto the body while skin is damp, immediately after showering or bathing. Daily supplements of at least 400 milligrams of vitamin E may also be helpful.

With psoriasis flaring up in cold and humid climates, intense sunlight and a UVB sunlamp aimed at the skin patches may alleviate some discomfort. When using this type of mechanism, don't forget to apply powerful sunscreen blocks to the psoriasis-free areas since ultraviolet Sun rays cause skin cancer. Do not use this type of therapy unless you have the go-ahead from a health care professional since it can sometimes do more harm than good.

Eczema

If you have itchy, dry, patchy red skin, you may be suffering from eczema. Keeping in mind that dry skin should be kept moist and well lubricated, the following suggestions will promote relief.

1. Use a cold-air humidifier as heat aggravates dry skin.
2. Avoid long, hot baths, which dry the skin, causing even more itching and flaking. Short, lukewarm baths with added essential oils can soften skin and provide relief, as do short, tepid showers.
3. Do not use scented soap, chemicals, or antibacterial agents like alpha-hydroxy, which aggravate the itch. If you must use soap, use a brand that is clear, or one which contains moisturizers such as lanolin, glycerine, palm oil, or coconut oil. In India, people routinely put coconut oil on their skin and hair as a protection from the scorching Sun. Try washing your face with lukewarm water, lightly patting it dry, followed by moisturizing cream or lotion such as Lubriderm, Keri, or Eucerin.

4. Avoid antiperspirants that contain metallic salts since they irritate sensitive skin.
5. Creams, ointments, and lotions that contain cortisone help to alleviate itching and redness. Hydrocortisone, the mildest form, is available over the counter.
6. Refrain from changing temperatures too rapidly. For instance, going from a warm room into cold air, or going from a cool room into a hot shower, can promote itching.
7. Clothing that touches your skin should be made of cotton or other natural fibers. Avoid wearing undergarments or inner garments made from wool or synthetics, to which you may be allergic or which can cause irritation and further itching. Even watchbands tainted with certain chemicals have been known to cause skin rashes.[10]

Following the above guidelines will help to relieve the discomfort or even prevent further outbreaks.

MINERAL SALT

The mineral salt related to Capricorn is calcium phosphate, which is needed to build strong bones and teeth as well as maintain blood vessels and digestive fluids. When this salt is lacking, there is a tendency toward dental troubles, skin irritations, and weak digestion, which may cause the formation of acid in the joints, leading to rheumatism and arthritis. Foods rich in calcium phosphate include cucumbers, spinach, lettuce, figs, plums, strawberries, almonds, lentils, whole wheat, barley, rye, fish, and milk.

AYURVEDA

Ruled by Saturn, Capricorn, an earth sign, falls under the auspices of sensitive Vata and practical Kapha. Vata-Kapha types have Kapha's easygoing and relaxed manner yet the resolve and gaseous, sensitive stomach found among Vata types. Capricorns are, however, not as slow-moving nor as plodding as Kapha Taurus and neither are they as nervous or sensitive as Vata Gemini or Virgo.

Although these two temperaments are opposite in that Vata is nervous and Kapha is placid, this combination provides inner stability, even-temperedness, and procrastination, yet quickness, efficiency, and anxiety when Capricorn needs to perform. Due to the sluggishness of the digestive system, a Vata-pacifying diet incorporating salty and sour foods like lemons, cheese, yogurt, tomatoes, plums, and vinegar stimulates the digestive system. Classified as sweet foods, warm milk, rice, hot bread with a little butter, porridge, honey, and sugar will settle your stomach and provide a satisfying breakfast. Don't forget that sweet foods also contribute to lethargy and accentuate a slow metabolism, so do not eat too much milk, bread, butter, or sugar. Do not eat bitter or astringent foods, which exacerbate gas pains and a sensitive stomach. (For more information on a Vata-pacifying diet, see Chapter 4.)

GEM AND COLOR THERAPY

If you were born between December 21 and December 31, your birthstone is the turquoise, a blue-green semiprecious stone common to Native American jewelry throughout the American Southwest. If you were born between January 1 and

January 19, your birthstone is the garnet, a dark red semi-precious stone associated with the Sun and energy. Garnets strengthen vitality, increase optimism, and can lighten Capricorn's dark moods. The metal ruling Capricorn is silver and ideally all your stones should be set in that metal. The colors associated with Saturn, Capricorn's ruling planet, are black and dark blue. Dark stones to which you respond include onyx, black sapphire, marcasite, and lapis lazuli.

Chapter 12

Aquarius the
Water Bearer

The High-Strung
Humanitarian

**AQUARIUS THE WATER BEARER
(JANUARY 20–FEBRUARY 18)
RULING PLANET: URANUS (SATURN CORULER)
ELEMENT: AIR
MODALITY: FIXED**

Positive Aquarius traits and concepts: social, people-oriented, generous, altruistic, intellectual, innovative, objective, idealistic, reformist, group-oriented, friendly, independent, freedom-loving, loyal, fair, and disciplined.

Negative Aquarius traits and concepts: eccentric, moody, high-strung, aloof, rebellious, impersonal, sharp-tongued, short attention span, neurotic, emotionally detached, inflexible, rigid, controlling, unpredictable, and finicky.

Parts of the body ruled by Aquarius include ankles, shins, veins, and circulatory system. Its ruling planet, Uranus, governs the nervous system and endocrine system.

Ailments include sprained ankle, nervous disorders, hormonal imbalances, hardening of the arteries, cramping, varicose veins, phlebitis, and hypertension.

Professions which focus on Aquarian inventiveness, idealism, group involvement, and humanitarian values include social worker, politician, teacher, group leader, psychologist, computer programmer, scientist, researcher, astronomer, and inventor.

AQUARIUS THE WATER BEARER:
REBELLIOUS SPIRIT LEADS YOU TO SUCCESS

Affiliation with organizations or causes that reflect strong ideals and social concerns is a hallmark of Aquarius the Water Bearer, a fixed air sign. Symbolized by the angel pouring water over the earth, Aquarians are outgoing, eccentric, high-strung individuals who crave constant excitement and intellectual stimulation. Although Aquarius represents friendship and brotherhood, you are often accused of being detached, insensitive, and more concerned with the plight of the world than with personal relationships. A walking contradiction, you are consumed with independence and truth, yet you have difficulty expressing deep feelings and detest being alone. For this reason you seek out those who share your political, social, and/or religious ideals.

Aquarians are natural rebels and the first to embrace lifestyle choices that are unorthodox, even radical. This may take the form of support groups, artistic collaborations, or even communal living. You are opinionated, unpredictable, and unconventional but very rarely will you strike out on your own. That is left to the fire signs. Aquarians, like all air signs, are concerned with opinions, support, and respect from family, friends, and colleagues.

Uranus, the ruler of Aquarius, was discovered in 1783 around the same time Benjamin Franklin discovered electricity. Due to this connection, Uranus-ruled Aquarians are said to have "electric," high-strung, anxious personalities and shine when they are surrounded by people they love and/or respect. On the other hand, you do not have a very long attention span when relating one-on-one. Nervous, fidgety, and irritable, especially if you must sit for long periods of time, you tend to make those around you uneasy as well.

Although you are humane, idealistic, empathetic, and will go to any lengths for close friends, you do have a dark side. With restrictive, fearful, and dutiful Saturn as the coruler of Aquarius, you often retreat for periods of time, shunning friends and loved ones. Since the struggle to keep your ideals alive requires that you face the world optimistically at all times, you vacillate between savoring your solitude and yearning for the crowd—earning the label of eccentricity.

Acting high-spirited when you are really down in the dumps creates inner tension which eventually finds a release—usually in the privacy of your own home and often directed at those you love. This low frustration tolerance, that is, an inability to react calmly in the face of crisis, results from lack of patience and not confronting obstacles head-on. Instead, you react in a frenzied manner, forgetting that if you approach things calmly and analytically, problems would be more easily resolved.

Fixed Aquarius may be gregarious, independent, and generous to a fault, but you are also stubborn, inflexible, and controlling. While you like excitement, your life is much too busy for spontaneity. Your calendar is often booked weeks in advance and once your schedule is planned, you are too inflexible to change midstream. Because of your overcommitted, chaotic lifestyle, you are chronically late and are known to regularly break appointments. Unfortunately, you do not always tolerate others who may do the same. Learning to organize time to allow quiet moments alone may help you to approach situations in a more level-headed fashion.

PHYSIOGNOMY AND BODY TYPE

Aquarians are characterized by nervous movements, verbosity, lively eyes, a strong nose, and a wide mouth. Marked by an air of nobility, the Aquarian face and expression often lack emotion.

Due to a high-strung nature, you are, more often than not, thin and wiry. There is usually something extraordinarily unique about your features or general appearance. Chances are you have a style of your own which assures that you will stand out in a crowd.

Individualistic and extremely spirited, Aquarians must guard against insomnia, hyperventilation, and panic attacks—each the result of nervous tension. Relaxation techniques, specific herbs, and exercises to prevent the onset of these ailments are discussed throughout this book. (See Chapter 4.)

Since you are mentally active, high-strung, and often anxiety-ridden, you will more than likely be prone to physical inactivity and hypertension—leading culprits of coronary artery disease. With Aquarius ruling the circulatory system, shins, calves, and ankles, you are a leading candidate for leg cramps and ankle sprains.

IMPROVING CIRCULATION

R uled by Aquarius, the circulatory system is comprised of the
cardiovascular system (*cardio* means "heart" and *vascular*
means "blood vessels") and the lymphatic system. Made up of arteries and veins, the vascular system transports blood and oxygen
throughout the body. If the vascular system is not able to dis-
tribute blood and oxygen efficiently, the result is poor circulation—a contributing factor in heart disease. Aside from
congenital weaknesses, factors that may contribute to circulatory
problems include hypertension (high blood pressure), high levels
of triglycerides and cholesterol in the bloodstream, smoking, excess weight, lack of exercise, water retention, and emotional
stress. Poor circulation also results in general lack of energy,
lower body heat, and more serious problems such as edema, varicose veins, phlebitis, clotting, and embolism.

To stimulate circulation, Aquarians are encouraged to engage
in strenuous exercise such as jogging, hiking, running, bicycling,
swimming, calisthenics, aerobics, or brisk walking for approximately thirty to sixty minutes at least three to four times a week.
These activities help burn calories and condition the heart and
lungs. Although it is unlikely that Aquarians will be drawn to
these competitive activities, active sports such as tennis, racquetball, soccer, basketball, and "touch" football are especially beneficial. Even moderate, regular physical activities like pleasure
walking, gardening, yard work, and dancing will help lower the
risk of heart disease.

Hypertension also puts you at risk for coronary ailments. It is
imperative to regulate hypertension by giving up cigarettes, eliminating salt, increasing potassium, losing weight, decreasing anxiety, and controlling anger. Drink six to eight glasses of water
daily, and take vitamin and mineral supplements if you do not

have the time to prepare nutritious meals at home. (See Chapters 4 and 10 on Gemini and Sagittarius for helpful hints on healthy fast food and nutritious dining out.)

CONQUER THE NICOTINE HABIT

Due to the high-strung, nervous traits of Aquarians, parting with nicotine will be difficult but it is a vice which must be halted immediately. If going cold turkey is not very appealing, consider attending Smokenders, a support group for smokers, or trying auriculotherapy, a technique which involves the placement of acupuncture needles in certain points on the ears. Combined with ongoing counseling sessions, this technique has proven effective in treating both nicotine and food addictions. Nicotine patches, available over the counter, allow the drug to penetrate the body in decreasing degrees until weaning is complete and the desire to smoke is completely eradicated.

Stress reduction techniques such as biofeedback, creative visualization, and acupuncture are highly recommended techniques to help you control irrational anger and temper tantrums, which elevate your blood pressure before they begin. (Read Chapter 6 for tips on lowering your blood pressure.)

GINKGO

An ancient Chinese remedy used for centuries to ease coughs, asthma, and inflammation due to allergies, ginkgo is a popular herb available in capsule form whose miraculous healing properties are finally getting the attention of the allopathic medical establishment. Although the ginkgo tree has been in existence for thousands of years, the extracts from its leaves are now readily available as a commercially prepared compound called Ginkgo Biloba. Commonly prescribed in Europe, Ginkgo Biloba has been praised for its ability to improve circulation and to effectively treat phlebitis (inflammation of a vein) and diabetic peripheral vascular disease by preventing blood clots.

Increasing the supply of blood traveling to the brain, ginkgo is also thought to improve memory, expand mental alertness, and thwart the onset of Alzheimer's disease. Studies have indeed shown that ginkgo users exhibit a significant improvement in mobility, orientation, communication, mental alertness, recent memory, and freedom from confusion. Because it also increases blood flow to the inner ear, it has even been used to treat vertigo and tinnitus (ringing in the ears). If you develop stomach upsets, nausea, and heartburn as a result of high doses of Ginkgo Biloba, reduce the dosage or take a break.

Ginkgo is also being tested to see whether it can provide relief to sufferers of depression, asthma, and other allergies. Its ability to strengthen the flow of blood by dilating arteries, veins, and capillaries is reputed to be a factor in slowing the aging process, though this has not yet been proven.

SWOLLEN ANKLES

One of the first signs of circulatory problems is swollen ankles, also known as edema. Although both temporary and chronic edema can occur throughout the body, Aquarians are especially prone to puffy ankles and swelling in the area directly below the knees. Temporary swelling caused by immobility can occur after sitting in an airplane, automobile, or bus for a long stretch, or even working at a desk for extended periods of time without elevating the legs. When you walk or run, leg muscles contract, compressing the vessels and promoting blood flow. When the muscles are not exercised, the blood accumulates and the fluid cannot easily move from the body tissues back to the blood vessels in the leg.

Hot weather also causes blood vessels to temporarily expand, allowing fluid to gather in the ankles, especially if there is an injury or poor circulation already present. (When I sprained my ankle several years ago, it remained swollen for longer than expected due to the hot, humid summer we had that year.)

Although temporary edema may simply be caused by immobility or injury, it could be a warning that circulation is not up to par. An overactive or underactive thyroid gland alters the concentration of protein in the blood, thereby preventing the free-flowing movement of blood. Inflammatory diseases such as rheumatoid arthritis and gout also cause swelling. If you have sudden, painful, and persistent swelling of both legs accompanied by shortness of breath and weight gain, it is important to see your physician immediately. Since the kidneys, liver, and heart affect blood pressure and fluid movement in and out of tissues, chronic edema can be indicative that these organs are somewhat afflicted.

Whether edema is temporary or chronic, steps to improve circulation like losing weight, exercising regularly, and elevating the legs may nip a potentially dangerous condition in the bud. Additionally, try to avoid basking in the sun, drink lots of fluid, and stay away from salty food. When you ingest more salt than you need, the body dilutes it by retaining fluids, leaving you even thirstier. Since an overage of salt elevates blood pressure, it is recommended that daily sodium intake should not exceed 3,000 milligrams. To maintain this level, season food with herbs and spices, read food labels to help track your sodium intake, and limit your consumption of salty foods. If these do not work, your physician may decide to prescribe diuretics.

HEALING HERBS

Don't be fooled by the fact that stinging nettles burn your hands when you come into contact with their prickly hairs, which contain a combination of histamine and formic acid. The amazing, medicinal properties of the flowers, leaves, and seeds of wild nettles have been used for centuries as an all-purpose panacea for kidney inflammation, hemorrhoids, rheumatism, gout, and allergies like hay fever. The leaves are rich in vitamins and minerals and should ideally be gathered before they blossom. They can be cooked like spinach or, more commonly, steeped as tea. When ingested, the leaves improve circulation and purify the blood. If you cannot find the leaves, nettles are also available in capsule form or in prepackaged tea. Nettles have proven useful in relieving shortness of breath, and function as an anti-inflammatory and blood purifier by ridding the body of fluids and reducing the tendency to edema.

Made from the berries of the elder plant, elderberry tonic and tea are powerful purgatives and anti-inflammatories which aid in the treatment of edema, gout, and eye inflammations by inducing sweating, increasing urine production, and clearing mucus from the lungs. Other herbs that successfully treat swellings include bryonia, dandelion, deadly nightshade, primrose, radish, saffron, and sarsaparilla. Carrot juice and asparagus can also control edema, gout, and rheumatism.

Because Aquarians are nervous and often insomniacs, any tranquilizing herb already discussed in this book will produce a calming effect. Bergamot, which creates the flavor in Earl Grey tea, is used to treat sleeplessness and is available as tea or an essential oil. Usually included in potpourri, it has a refreshing and relaxing scent. Borage, a common garden herb taken as an infusion, contains potassium and calcium. It is an antidepressant and tension reliever reputed to help heal sprains and stimulate the heart. If you do sprain your ankle, try Rescue Remedy (see Chapter 2) or Rhus. Tox., a homeopathic tincture which will reduce the swelling immediately.

Dandelion, used for tea, wine, juice, and as a coffee substitute, contains calcium and iron, and has also been used to treat poor circulation, bowel inflammation, and stomach disorders. Red clover, chamomile, and valerian tea tranquilize and strengthen the nervous system and guarantee an uninterrupted night's sleep when taken before retiring. Added to bathwater, rosemary oil reduces hypertension, stimulates the circulation, and increases body heat. Bilberry leaves are said to reduce varicose veins, hyssop regulates blood pressure, and caraway strengthens sprained limbs.

Hawthorn, an herb whose berries produce a liquid extract, has been recognized for its ability to increase the muscular action of the heart, help dilate the coronary vessels, and improve the blood's ability to utilize oxygen. Taken as a tonic by swallowing five to twelve drops three times a day, or by adding two tablespoons of its buds to one cup of boiling water twice a day, hawthorn helps to ease insomnia, angina, hypertension, and other circulatory disorders. If you are a Leo or Aquarius and feel that you could have a proclivity toward hypertension, you may wish to use this cardiac tonic. While hawthorn is considered safe and effective, it is not a substitute for heart medication. If you wish to use the herb alongside your present medication, first see if your doctor approves.

ANKLE SPRAINS

Since Aquarians are prone to ankle sprains and swelling, it is very important to wear supportive shoes, walk slowly, and watch where you are going. If you fall, twist, or sprain your ankle, be certain to elevate your leg right away, place an ice pack on it, and reach for ibuprofen or another anti-inflammatory to reduce the swelling. If pain persists, see a physician immediately as it may be necessary to immobilize your leg. Do not treat a sprain lightly nor assume that it will heal quickly. Be aware that a sprain is a deep-tissue injury that can weaken your leg for quite some time.

VARICOSE VEINS

One of the most common vascular problems, varicose veins are characterized by abnormally enlarged and swollen veins most commonly found near the surface of the leg. Varicose veins usually surface with age, when the valves in the veins which normally keep blood flowing from the legs back to the heart fail, causing the blood to flow downward, where it gathers in pools, affecting general circulation.

Varicose veins are the result of damage to deep veins in the legs due to injury, blood clots or inflammation. The symptoms include pain and swelling of the surface veins, which are usually small and not associated with the type of blood clots that can travel to the heart or lungs, causing an obstruction (embolism). There may be inflammation, but the clot does not pose a serious threat to your health as long as it remains on the surface. If varicose veins progress, however, the skin covering the vein may become dry, irritated, and itchy, ultimately resulting in phlebitis, a serious complication of varicose veins, characterized by further reddening and swelling of the veins, increased pulse rate, slight fever, and pain in the afflicted area. Eventually a clot could escape from the venous wall and lodge in a blood vessel. Sponging the legs with cold water and cool compresses with the essential oils of cypress, rosemary, and peppermint may bring relief to swollen veins. If your symptoms worsen, consult your physician, who will either inject medication directly into the veins or opt for laser therapy.

There are no specific instructions on how to avoid this condition but there are suggestions as to how to reduce some of the risk factors. While pregnancy does not cause varicose veins per se, many women who are expecting develop them because of the increased pressure on the pelvic veins and the hormonal changes that occur during this period. The greatest risk factor is having a parent with varicose veins. Other factors include nicotine, obesity, tight clothing, and sedentary occupation, which requires sitting or standing for prolonged periods of time.

If you are at risk for developing varicose veins, refrain from sitting for prolonged periods of time, and make sure that you get plenty of exercise. Walking, running, cycling, and swimming are ways to improve muscle tone and circulation. If you must sit without a break, whenever possible uncross and elevate your legs above chest level using pillows or a chair. Support hose can also relieve the pressure. Vitamins B (especially niacin) and C are necessary for the maintenance of strong blood vessels and prevention of blood clots. Vitamin E helps to dilate blood vessels, improve circulation, and may reduce susceptibility to varicose veins.

To foster circulation in your legs, avoid very hot baths, which can break up veins under your skin. Massaging your legs daily from your toes to your thighs with vitamin E oil, a combination of lemon and lavender oil, or any other warm massage oil can improve circulation. The oil should either be at room temperature or slightly warm.

1. Sit on the floor with your legs outstretched, bending them at the knees.

2. Applying oil to a leg, briskly rub the front and back of your lower leg in an up-and-down motion. This warms your leg and increases circulation.

3. First squeeze each part of the muscles extending down the calf and afterward use circular movements up and down the leg between the ankle and the knee.

4. Use small, circular motions around the kneecap and over the knee.

5. Lower your leg slightly and rub oil on the area between the knee and the thigh.

6. Using both hands, one behind the other, move your fingertips from the knee to the thigh and back down to the knee, squeezing each area.

7. Using your knuckles, knead the leg from the knee up to the groin, encompassing the thigh. This will create friction, warm the leg, and increase blood flow.

8. After you are finished with both legs, stretch them directly in front of you, pointing and flexing the feet.

After the massage, try to sit, if possible, for twenty minutes to a half-hour with your feet elevated. Massage is a wonderful tool for stimulating blood flow. You don't need to be a professional. You can be your own masseuse and practice self-massage by following the above steps.

With Aquarius ruling the shins, the ankles, and the lower leg, you will likely be prone to leg cramps. If you are exercising or walking when this occurs, stop immediately. The pain may be gone as quickly as it came. Cramps usually occur at night or after activity but are also common to people with poor circulation and arteriosclerosis. Cramping can be problematic at any age, especially if a hereditary factor is present or you do not take proper care of yourself.

The first line of defense is applying ice on the affected area at twenty-minute intervals throughout the day. After some time you may wish to switch to warm compresses, baths, or a heating pad. Any over-the-counter anti-inflammatory will help reduce pain. Raising your leg higher than your heart is recommended.

Frequent cramping may be caused by deficiencies in calcium, thiamine, pantothenic acid, biotin, magnesium, or sodium. Vitamin C is necessary to ensure proper circulation and helps ease pain in the muscles and joints. Protein will hasten the healing process.

YOGA ASANAS

PADAHASTASANA (LEG CLASP)

Padahastasana (Leg Clasp) is a simple yoga exercise that helps the knees, calves, and heels. It is especially suited for firming calves and thighs.

1. Stand upright with your heels together.
2. Slowly bend forward from the hips, keeping your legs straight.
3. Bring arms back and clasp your hands behind your knees.
4. Slowly bend your head toward your knees and torso as far as you can go.
5. Hold this position for ten minutes.
6. Straighten to an upright position and relax briefly before repeating the exercise again.

AROMATHERAPY AND ESSENTIAL OILS

Jasmine, marigold, orange blossom, and lavender oils are each equally helpful for relieving anxiety, insomnia, and nervous tension especially if you add ten drops of your favorite scent to a warm bath before bedtime. These oils can also be inhaled or massaged onto the abdomen (solar plexus). Marjoram, chamomile, sandalwood, lavender, or ylang-ylang added to the bath, inhaled, massaged onto the abdomen, or used in an incense burner or vaporizer helps depression. Orange blossom and rose, two extraordinarily fragrant scents, can ease irritability and moodiness simply because they evoke serenity and inner peace. To improve the unsightliness of varicose veins caused by broken capillaries, apply ointments or creams which contain peppermint, lavender, and lemon oil for use during the day, and neroli, rose, and chamomile for night applications. When added to the bath or inhaled, juniper and rosemary oil are both recommended to stimulate circulation.

AYURVEDA

Since Aquarius is ruled by Saturn and Uranus, two Vata planets, it is no wonder that those born under this air sign are high-strung, nervous, and often stressed. Like most other Vata types, Aquarians have very delicate nervous systems, finding it difficult to relax and enjoy life by taking it one day at a time. Their minds work overtime and, as a result, frequently suffer from bouts of insomnia. A worrisome, anxious, and pessimistic approach to life is not uncommon to Aquarians or anyone who resonates to the Vata temperament.

It is most therapeutic for Aquarians to exercise regularly, eat three square meals a day, and go to sleep at the same time each evening. Stimulants should be avoided at all costs, especially late in the afternoon or early evening. Getting a professional massage is highly recommended for Vata types whose main problem is the inability to relax and slow down. To this end, meditation is an absolute must, even though quieting the mind will be extremely challenging.

A diet which pacifies Vata is a necessity for Aquarians. Because Vata dosha is cold and dry, it is important to consume warm foods like soups, stews, hot-baked bread, and hearty casseroles. Because Aquarians tend to be thin and burn up fat with their quick metabolism, adding warm, melted butter to your food (in moderation of course) is soothing for Vata types, especially since they are usually thin with lots of nervous energy. Salty, sweet, and sour foods are also recommended (see Chapter 4). Because your stomach is sensitive, try to eat in peaceful surroundings, and be sure you eat slowly, and sit down for your entire meal. Eating and running simply will not do. Start the day with hot cereal, especially cream of rice or wheat, or anything with added milk. Pasta dishes, rice, and lentils are all good for the dinner menu. Drinking warm milk before going to bed will help you sleep through the night—something Aquarians generally miss.

MINERAL SALT

The mineral salt associated with Aquarius is sodium chloride (NaCl), otherwise known as common table salt. Sodium chloride helps to maintain water content throughout the body. Eliminated from the body quickly, salt must be replaced. Although a deficiency will cause runny nose, watery eyes, dry skin and mucous membranes, do not add table salt to food as this will exacerbate water retention and hypertension, to which Aquarians are already prone. Instead eat more spinach, cabbage, lettuce, cucumbers, lentils, figs, strawberries, apples, carrots, radishes, and chestnuts—all foods high in sodium chloride.

GEM AND COLOR THERAPY

If your birthday is between January 20 and January 31, your birthstone is the garnet, a dark red stone that is also associated with the Sun, which rules Leo—a sign which, like Aquarius, is prone to circulatory ailments. If you are born between February 1 and 18, your birthstone is the amethyst, a lovely purple stone renowned for its healing ability, especially in the treatment of migraine headaches. Other stones that stimulate the circulation, reduce hypertension, and invigorate the heart muscle include coral, carnelian, and bloodstone. The colors governed by Aquarius are red, which symbolizes the flow of blood, and black, associated with Saturn, the coruler of Aquarius. Sitting in the Sun, bathing under a red light, wearing red clothes, and buying freshly cut red roses all act to restore vitality and increase blood flow.

Chapter 13

Pisces the Fish

Keep Your Feet Planted
Firmly on the Ground

PISCES THE FISH (FEBRUARY 19–MARCH 20)
RULING PLANET: Neptune (coruler Jupiter)
ELEMENT: Water
MODALITY: Mutable

Positive Pisces traits and concepts: imaginative, creative, good-hearted, sensitive, sympathetic, generous, sensual, helpful, dutiful, flexible, open-minded, compassionate, romantic, humble, emotional, and intuitive.

Negative Pisces traits and concepts: addictive, escapist, indulgent, deceitful, dishonest, lazy, indecisive, low self-esteem, insecure, careless, vague, confused, impractical, fearful, and shy.

Parts of the body ruled by Pisces include the toes, feet, lymph nodes, pituitary, and pineal glands. Its ruling planet, Neptune, governs the lymphatic system.

Ailments include swollen ankles, obesity, alcoholism, drug addiction, poor circulation, water retention, glandular disorders, and mucus in the lungs.

Professions which appeal to Pisces' creativity, imagination, love of fantasy, altruism, and sensitivity include artist, dancer, painter, poet, actor, illustrator, nurse, medical personnel, photographer, clergy, and restaurateur.

Pisces the Fish:
You Have What It Takes to Make Your Dreams Come True

Pisces, a mutable water sign symbolized by two fish swimming in opposite directions, is emotional, imaginative, and sensitive, yet naive and extremely impressionable. Highly sympathetic and compassionate, you often overlook your own capabilities and rely on friends and lovers to provide you with the confidence you lack. While you go out of your way to be kind and generous, especially to those less fortunate, you struggle to find the self-assurance, determination, and aggression necessary to face the hard, cruel world. There's no doubt that your indecisiveness and timidity are responsible for a few personal and professional opportunities falling by the wayside. It's not that you lack strong ideals and opinions. It's just that once you encounter adversity, your insecurity and self-effacement prevent you from placing value on what you believe.

Not only is Pisces easily hurt by remarks which would slide off someone else's back, but decision making is especially excruciating since you always consider the feelings of others before your own. While you are keenly aware that hemming, hawing, and endless vacillation irritate others, it is almost impossible for you to take a step forward until everyone is happy—an impossible task. Nevertheless, you are more than relieved when the decision-making process is taken out of your hands. If you do wind up in a position of authority, there is always the likelihood you will be taken advantage of unless you stand up and be counted. To successfully work with others, you must develop confidence in your point of view and develop a tougher skin. Unfortunately, the idea of confrontation scares you beyond belief.

Assertiveness training is merely one form of therapy which can help you to stand firm behind your opinions. Since you are intuitive rather than analytical and methodical, this type of therapy, which can be done privately or in a group, could teach you to trust your instincts and act on them.

In the end, you would rather be left alone to work at your own pace and to follow your impulses. Lack of discipline and an inability to sit still for long periods of time make it difficult, but not impossible, for you to direct your creativity to a successful conclusion. Once you do, however, admiration for your amazing artistry, imagination, and spontaneity is usually forthcoming and immensely rewarding.

The need to be loved is so overpowering that it makes you unnecessarily dependent and insecure. When confronted with problems, you tend to take the road of least resistance. Naturally shy, apprehensive, and fearful, you will sacrifice your own needs to make someone happy and/or avoid confrontation. The empathy and unselfishness which guide your behavior are so overwhelming that you literally give others "the shirt off your back." Learn to say no once in a while. You'll be surprised how good it feels, once you conquer the guilt which guides many of your actions.

Whenever possible, you will offer financial and/or emotional support to anyone in need. If you have improved the life of even one individual, you feel fulfilled, but as a result, you often confuse sympathy with love. The belief that emotional strength and/or monetary assistance are the means to attract others can deter you from developing a strong sense of self and lead you deeper into destructive relationships.

Truly benevolent and compassionate, you are oftentimes compelled to sacrifice your own agendas to win love and affection. Due to misplaced sympathy, you attract needy people, thus forming hopeless, codependent relationships. (See Chapter 8.) Should your partner recover, the relationship often disintegrates since it has been based not on love but on the need to help and support. Sensitive, sensual, creative, and loving, you must accept that someone will love you for yourself and not for what you have to give. The helping professions, volunteering, and charity work each provides an outlet for your compassion and sense of duty. Ultimately, you will no longer need to magnify these in your personal relationships.

Incredibly kind, gentle, affable, and liked by everyone you meet, sensual Pisceans like yourself are usually motivated by the sheer need to feel good. Since you simply want to love and be loved, feeling good can mean being paid attention to, sexual enjoyment, or the elation that comes when you feel you are helping someone get back on his feet. It is necessary to develop perseverance and resilience to bounce back after disappointments and losses.

It is vital for you to recognize your own self-worth, and to realize that you deserve happiness and serenity. Due to your fertile imagination, spirituality, and belief in the paranormal, creative visualization exercises and hypnotherapy will work especially well.

PHYSIOGNOMY AND BODY TYPE

Your face is usually round with large, saucer-shaped eyes, full cheeks, pointed chin, and a graceful neck. Your lips are thick and sensual. With an enjoyment of sensual pleasures and a tendency to retain fluids, you can easily be overweight. Once you feel good, you don't always know when to stop. Since Pisceans are susceptible to alcohol and drugs, you should be cautious when imbibing at a festive event. Even a single drink may be one too many. This sensitivity can also manifest as an allergy to antibiotics, especially penicillin. If so, be certain to obtain a medical-alert bracelet inscribed with that vital information.

You may, in fact, be allergic to chocolate, strawberries, nuts, dust, and/or cats. Conditions like hay fever and asthma are also not uncommon among Pisceans. Many of these allergic reactions often manifest when you are a child, and either diminish in severity or completely disappear once you reach adulthood. Don't be surprised, however, if these allergies resurface after the age of fifty, or when you've had too much to drink.

THE LYMPHATIC SYSTEM

Ruled by Pisces, the lymphatic system, a group of organs and vessels which make up the majority of our body's immune system, is closely linked to the Aquarius-ruled circulatory system. It's no wonder that Pisceans and Aquarians are both prone to swollen ankles and poor circulation (Aquarius rules the ankles and Pisces retains water).

The lymphatic system (and the organs which comprise it) is the body's first line of defense for blocking toxins from the bloodstream. When an infection is present, its glands, the most prominent of which are the lymph nodes in the neck and armpits, can become enlarged, even painful. Once the infection is gone, the swelling subsides. The more stress to the body, the harder and longer the lymph nodes must work to return to their normal state.

Other factors that weaken the lymphatic system so it is incapable of fighting disease are allergies, poor diet, tight clothing, and an accumulation of excess hormones, resulting in a variety of disorders. These include skin lesions, chronic sinusitis, ear problems, loss of balance, headaches, excess sweating, puffy eyes, fatigue, and edema.

Since Pisceans are prone to water retention, many of the diuretic herbs and remedies mentioned throughout this book can be utilized to eliminate excess fluids. (See Chapter 12.) Alfalfa, added to salads as sprouts or ingested as tea, is a great diuretic which can aid Pisces' struggle to overcome water retention, weight gain, and poor circulation.

Highly creative but ultimately lazy, your love of gymnastics, figure skating, and all forms of dancing (from modern to jazz to folk) can provide the exercise you need and the creativity you crave. Swimming, water skiing, boating, and other water sports also appeal to Pisceans who, like Cancerians, feel at home in or around water. (See Chapter 5 for hydrotherapy techniques.) Your lack of mental toughness may make competitive sports a bit overwhelming. If you train extremely hard and develop a firm belief in yourself, it is not impossible to cultivate the ability to function under great pressure and, most important, to withstand rejection. A support system of family, friends, and physical trainers can help to remind you of your talents and strengths.

ALCOHOLISM AND ADDICTION

Due to emotional vulnerability and general insecurity, you experience great difficulty rebounding after a disappointment or rejection. Whereas many people can simply chalk up letdowns to experience and move forward, you do not always possess the inner resolve to accomplish this and are quick to label yourself a failure. If immediate reassurance, approval, and comfort are not forthcoming from a partner or friend after a setback, it is likely you will seek instant gratification by overspending, overeating, drinking, or even through drug addiction. While an occasional excess may not prove harmful, your lack of willpower puts you at great risk for dependency and indulgent, self-destructive behavior.

With water, fluids, and escapism falling under the auspices of your ruling planet, Neptune, the Greco-Roman lord of the sea, you may be prone to alcoholism, a chronic, progressive, and potentially fatal disease characterized by both physical and emotional dependency on alcohol. Although there is disagreement as to whether alcoholism is hereditary or learned, most experts concur that, whether biological or psychological, a predisposition to alcohol addiction is genuine. Those with this disease develop drinking habits which are completely uncontrollable, and even one drink will trigger the psychological and physical need for more.

If you cannot get through the day without a drink, and if you find that two or three drinks are needed to produce the effect formerly achieved by one, you may be on the road to alcoholism if not already a full-fledged alcoholic. One way to assess whether you have a problem is if you experience even minor psychological and physical withdrawal symptoms if you are alcohol-free for even a few hours.

Psychological dependence occurs when you are completely preoccupied with how and when you will get the next drink. It spawns apathy, chronic lateness, irritability, anger, and insensitive, even mean, behavior. You often cancel appointments, and your work performance steadily declines. In the advanced stages of alcoholism, there is short-term memory loss and blackouts, which can be as short as a few minutes or can last for hours. If chunks of your daily life disappear from your memory, it is a clear indication that alcohol problems exist, and you should seek help. In addition to the long-term psychological ramifications of alcohol abuse, the physical effects of full-blown alcoholism include cramps, vomiting, elevated blood pressure, sweating, dilated pupils, insomnia, and, at an advanced stage, convulsions. If you can abstain for two or three days, the symptoms may subside. Without willpower or the support of therapy or a twelve-step program, it is more than likely that you will reach for the bottle and begin the cycle again.

Long-term alcohol abuse is considered a factor in the onset of diabetes, kidney ailments, heart disease, ulcers, gastritis, and, in the extreme, cirrhosis of the liver, a condition which builds up after many years and results in major destruction of liver cells and a buildup of scar tissue. (See Chapter 10.)

You may be in complete denial about your problem. According to Alcoholics Anonymous, the following warning signs can alert you to a potential drinking problem.

1. Have you ever decided to stop drinking for a week or so, but only lasted for a couple of days?
2. Do you wish people would mind their own business about your drinking and stop telling you what to do?
3. Have you ever switched from one kind of drink to another in the hope that this would keep you from getting drunk?

4. Have you had to have an eye-opener upon awakening during the past year?
5. Do you need a drink to get started, or to stop shaking?
6. Do you envy people who can drink without getting into trouble?
7. Have you had problems connected with drinking during the past year?
8. Has your drinking caused trouble at home?
9. Do you ever try to get "extra" drinks at a party because you do not get enough?
10. Do you tell yourself you can stop drinking any time you want to, even though you keep getting drunk when you don't mean to?
11. Have you missed days of work or school because of drinking?
12. Do you have "blackouts"?
13. Have you ever felt that your life would be better if you did not drink?

If you answered yes to at least four of the aforementioned questions, think twice before you take your next drink. You could be suffering from alcoholism—a chronic yet manageable disease.

TREATMENT

The standard treatment for alcoholism is nothing less than complete abstinence. Once you have come to the end of your rope and have made the decision to seek help, it is imperative to obtain counseling and join a support group such as Alcoholics Anonymous (AA). This twelve-step, self-help group has enabled thousands upon thousands of alcoholics to manage their ailment and resume living normal lives. Acutely aware that most alcoholics suffer from shame, self-recrimination, and the fear of discovery, AA provides anonymity in a completely supportive atmosphere—just as its name suggests. Attending meetings will help you understand the nature of your ailment and improve your self-esteem so you can confront life situations without reaching for the bottle. Support groups enable you to find a sponsor, who will guide you through the twelve-step recovery process and on whom you can rely for advice and the benefit of his/her own experience in battling this disease.

If you are recovering from alcoholism, it is necessary to reintroduce nutrients into your system which have probably been depleted. These include supplements or food containing zinc (including meats, poultry, fish, whole-grain products, brewer's yeast, wheat bran, and pumpkin seeds), vitamin B, which strengthens the nervous system, and vitamin C. Because low blood sugar is a by-product of alcoholism it is also a good idea to increase the intake of complex carbohydrates, including whole grains, fresh vegetables and fruits, and all sugars and white bread. Herbs and relaxation techniques can help you avoid withdrawal symptoms, which include anxiety, nervousness, and insomnia. Catnip, chamomile, peppermint, skullcap, and hypericum are all recommended for depression. Burdock root and echinacea are very good purifiers. Kudzu root was discovered by Chinese doctors as a means to reduce the appetite for alcohol.

Combined with counseling and lifestyle changes, acupuncture and auriculotherapy (acupuncture around the ears) in particular have proven very effective in treating nicotine, food, and alcohol addictions.

While excessive behavior patterns are often rooted in a lack of self-esteem and the need for instant gratification, alcohol abuse, compulsive eating, and drug dependency may also be habits to which you are genetically predisposed.* Psychological addictions, such as compulsive spending and gambling, are frequently as uncontrollable as those which are physical and withdrawal just as excruciating. There are twelve-step programs, support groups, rehabilitation programs, and therapy available for each of these addictions. The common thread is a desire to conquer these destructive behavior patterns and, most important, discover or rediscover your own self-worth.

HYPNOTHERAPY

Because Pisceans are impressionable and trusting, hypnotherapy, a form of hypnosis that relies on the power of suggestion, may be the treatment of choice in treating addictions and improving low self-esteem, often the underlying cause of those behavior problems. While hypnosis alone induces a light trance during which time you receive a suggestion, hypnotherapy involves utilizing the therapeutic process while you are in the trance state. Hypnotherapy has been successful in treating psychological, emotional, and physical conditions since patients display less fear and resistance in a semiconscious state and are, therefore, more receptive to new ways of dealing with emotions, mind, or body.

Because you are intuitive and trusting, this therapy can be very effective in helping to conquer deep fears and even phobias not uncommon among Pisceans due to insecurities and a fertile imagination. Some of these may include fear of the dark, hypochondria, vertigo (fear of heights), and agoraphobia (fear of leaving the house). As a child, you may have had terrible night-

---

* Researchers have long believed that, due to a genetic factor, some people cannot recognize when they have had enough food and, therefore, overeat. Some people may also have food allergies which cause them to gorge.

mares and, even now, have vivid, unforgettable dreams. Through the hypnotherapist's suggestions during one-on-one therapy sessions and, at your leisure, with audiotapes, the messages which he or she conveys can actually work wonders. Your receptivity will enable you to embrace other therapeutic techniques such as dream therapy, where you record and revisit dreams to understand yourself, and regression, which forces you to relive and come to terms with childhood traumas.

Creative expression is by far the best antidote for fighting addiction and regaining faith in your abilities. Whenever you are disappointed and feel the urge to indulge, turn to art, music, or dancing—fulfilling, enjoyable pastimes to keep you on the straight and narrow.

ANEMIA

Characterized by constant fatigue and dizziness, anemia, or iron-poor blood, is a condition that arises when oxygenated blood is not transported to the body's cells by the hemoglobin, a combination of iron, copper, and protein present in red blood cells. Symptoms include general weakness, fatigue, paleness, brittle nails, loss of appetite, bruising, and abdominal pain. While iron, protein, copper, folic acid, and vitamins B_6, B_{12}, and C are all necessary for the formation of red blood cells, iron deficiency is the main cause of anemia.

To remedy anemia, the first rule of thumb is to supplement the diet with iron to build up the quality of the blood, thus increasing resistance to stress and disease. Iron supplements are available in capsules or by eating leafy green vegetables (especially spinach), tomatoes, raisins, whole grains, and legumes. One of the best sources of iron is liver, which is also high in protein, phosphorus, copper, and vitamins A, B, C, and D. Like all organ meat, however, it is an extremely high-cholesterol food and, therefore, should not be eaten more than once a week. It is recommended that you add the other iron-rich foods to your diet and snack on raisins from time to time.

Copper, also necessary for proper bone formation, can help prevent anemia by facilitating iron absorption. The best sources of copper are liver, whole-grain products, almonds, seafood, green leafy vegetables, and dried legumes.

In addition to nutritional therapy, take alfalfa, which contains iron, calcium, phosphorus, potassium, chlorine, sodium, silicon, magnesium, protein, and vitamins A, B, D, E, and K. A blood tonic and purifier, mineral-rich nettles are also used to treat anemia. Since nettle tea is a popular beverage, nettles, high in vitamin C, are readily available in health food stores.

FOOT MASSAGE

Since the feet contain a complete network of nerve endings, foot massage is a wonderful way to soothe the entire body at the end of a long day. Ask your partner to give you a relaxing foot massage, or self-massage your feet using the following guidelines.

1. Begin by rubbing warm oil onto a foot, which is usually the driest area of your body. Be certain that the oil is lukewarm or at room temperature.
2. Enclose the foot between both hands, then slowly slide your hands off the foot coming forward to the toes. Repeat this movement four or five times.
3. Using your thumbs, circle the ankle.
4. With your thumbs moving in little circles, go from the ankle to the toes. Repeat three or four times.

5. With a circular movement, rub each toe individually, ending by rotating each first clockwise then counterclockwise.

6. Gently pull each toe using your thumb and forefinger. You may hear a cracking noise when tension is released.

7. Move down the sole of your foot from the toes to your heel.

8. Once again, with your palms enclosing your foot, rub vigorously to create friction.

9. End by rotating the foot, pointing the toes, and then flexing the ankle.

10. Wrap the foot with a towel so that it is warm.

11. Repeat this exercise on the other foot.[11]

After a massage, further soothe your feet for fifteen minutes in a footbath to which lemon, sage, and/or peppermint essential oils have been added.

FOOT REFLEXOLOGY

If you discover that any of the areas on the feet are painful when pressure is applied, a reflexology massage might be the next step. In contrast to relaxing foot massage, foot reflexology, a system by which pressure is applied to the points on the feet that correspond to body parts and organs, is both a diagnostic and healing tool. (See Fig 13.1.) In the course of a foot massage, a reflexologist can, for example, discover that the kidneys are weak if the point on the foot relating to them is sensitive and/or painful when kneaded.

Although there are reflexology points throughout the body, the feet are most commonly used since they contain approximately seven thousand nerve endings which correspond to different areas throughout the body. Applying pressure to these points on the feet relieves tension and helps heal the corresponding area of the body by clearing obstruction and easing pain. If you have a headache, for example, work the toes. Reflexology activates the nervous system and stimulates the lymphatic system's healing power by opening the flow of lymph fluid into damaged areas.[12]

Since Pisceans are notorious for having cold, dry feet, use foot powder or vitamin E oil during the winter when the soles of the feet get extremely dry. Athlete's foot, a fungus infection which appears in the form of inflammation, rash, or scaly skin, is a common Piscean ailment. Make sure you do not go barefoot in locker rooms, steam baths, health clubs, or public bathrooms since fungi are easily transmitted under warm, moist conditions. Change socks several times a day, use foot powder, and take vitamins A, C, and E for the general health of your skin. Don't wear tight shoes and try not to go barefoot, even at home. Essential oils will keep the joints supple and prevent flaking especially in the winter.

TAI CHI CHUAN FOR PISCES

Because you are gentle, sensitive, and dislike aggression, tai chi chuan (commonly called tai chi), which consists of long, flowing, gentle movements in place of sharp, aggressive motions, is the perfect form of mind-body meditation. A centuries-old Chinese discipline, tai chi was, like any form of martial arts, originally conceived as a set of offensive and defensive maneuvers concentrating on quickness, vitality, and flexibility, but has evolved into a series of gentle exercises utilized to attain self-control, improve concentration, and achieve discipline. Like acupuncture, tai chi promotes the flow of chi—life energy—and replaces stiffness with flexibility and good body coordination.

While these qualities explain why tai chi originally worked as a method of self-defense, this series of movements improves circulation, limbers the body, tones muscles, improves physical fitness, and increases blood circulation. As a form of meditation which relaxes the body and mind, tai chi promotes mental tranquillity, strengthens the nervous system, and helps release tension.

Tai chi is comprised of a series of postures that flow and connect so the body and mind work harmoniously. With both feet on the ground, spine held upright, and knees slightly bent, the tai chi practitioner sways from side to side as if in a slow-motion dance, using the arms to guide each movement. This left-to-right motion exemplifies the Chinese principal of yin-yang, which represents the duality of night and day, active and passive, male and female. Each step, originally adapted from the natural movements of animals and birds, has a different poetic name, like "White Crane spreads its wings," which accurately describes the particular movement.

Like Hatha yoga's Sun Salutation, tai chi is traditionally practiced outdoors at sunrise to greet the dawning of the new day. Routinely performed, tai chi chuan can provide energy, discipline, and the concentration you need to perform your daily activities. Once all the postures are learned, they should be done slowly, softly, and gracefully as one long, continuous movement, paying attention to the position of the body and natural breathing rhythm. Tai chi will help you feel centered as the movements are geared to bring you back to Earth—the core of gravity. Even if you do not learn the entire series of movements and/or cannot practice this activity outside or at sunrise, try to set aside at least twenty minutes several times a week to practice tai chi.

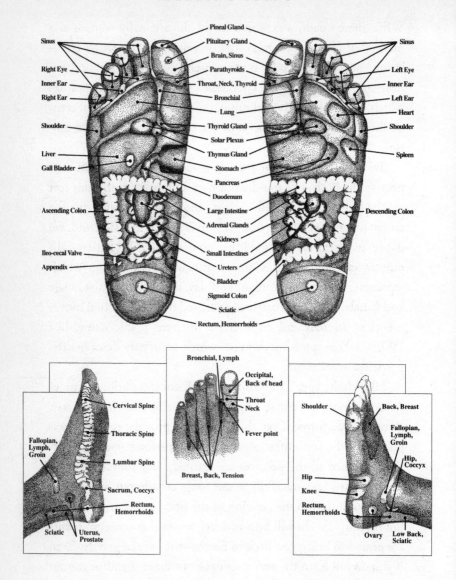

FIGURE 13.1 REFLEXOLOGY

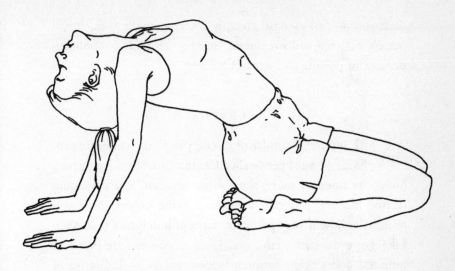

FIGURE 13.2 BACKWARD BEND

BACKWARD BEND (FIG 13.2)

Backward Bend is a yoga posture which enhances the flexibility of the feet, ankles, and toes as follows:

1. Take out a mat on which you can rest.
2. Place your knees together and rest your buttocks on your heels.
3. Extend your arms behind you and place the palms on the floor. Your arms must be parallel with the fingers pointing ahead of you.
4. As in the illustration, slowly lower your head back, arch your spine inward, and hold that position for about ten minutes, continuing to breathe steadily.

If you do this exercise properly several times a week, it will not only stretch and strengthen your legs and feet but will improve your posture and sense of balance.

AYURVEDA

With Jupiter as coruler of Pisces, you fit the complete profile of a Kapha personality. Characterized by sleeping long hours, retention of water, sluggish metabolism, and a tranquil, relaxed manner, you can range from being overweight if you overeat, or lithe if your particular form of indulgence is alcohol. Like Taureans, Cancerians, and Librans, you too are prone to puffiness and ringlets forming below your eyes—indicative of fluids not being properly released by the body. When you are functioning at your optimum, you are extremely patient, generous, and productive. But when out of balance there is a tendency toward lethargy, laziness, and poor circulation, resulting in edema and cold hands and feet.

To speed up your metabolic rate, Pisceans, like all Kapha types, must stimulate the system by changing dietary habits and embarking on a regular workout routine. Foods that must be completely avoided (at least until you have reestablished a sense of balance) include sweet foods such as sugar, honey, rice, milk, cream, and butter; and sour foods such as lemons, cheese, yogurt, tomatoes, grapes, plums, and vinegar. Due to their heaviness, all wheat products, including bread, pasta, and most cereals, which induce even more lethargy, should be eliminated from the diet. In addition, cut down on salt and salty foods since they promote water retention.

To stimulate the metabolism include pungent foods like cayenne, chili peppers, onions, garlic, radishes, ginger, and curry; bitters such as endive, chicory, romaine lettuce, and spinach; and beans, lentils, apples, pears, cabbage, broccoli, cauliflower, and potatoes, which fall under the category of astringent. Since they are considered "light" foods, they promote better digestion and, at the same time, curb the appetite. Instead of three meals, Kapha types are better off eating five or six smaller meals throughout the day.

As already stated, undisciplined Pisceans are likely to gravitate toward aquatic sports, dancing, skating, or gymnastics. Running, aerobics, and weight lifting are also recommended. Since Kapha is a cold dosha, you crave warmth and, therefore, prefer activities that can also be done indoors. (For more information about Kapha dosha, see Chapter 3.)

HERBAL REMEDIES FOR PISCEAN AILMENTS

Hyssop, a popular member of the mint family, has been used since biblical times as a digestive aid. In the form of tea, it helps to relieve colds, coughs, hoarseness, and sore throats. It is also used externally to treat sores and bruises. Kelp, which contains iron, can be taken as a supplement to treat anemia. Bilberry counteracts water retention, chicory reduces mucus, eyebright helps conjunctivitis, and horseradish is recommended for glandular problems.

AROMATHERAPY AND ESSENTIAL OILS

As you are sensual and extremely sensitive to smells, sweet essential oils such as rose, jasmine, and orange blossom are great mood elevators especially when you are down in the dumps and feeling insecure. To perfume the room, buy or make your own potpourri, or bouquet, from an array of fragrances which you find especially pleasing. To make potpourri, begin by crumbling together dried bunches of flowers and herbs. Add essential oils of your choice so that the combination of scents permeates the room. For a fresh and light aroma, try lemon, coriander, vetiver, and melissa; for a warm and spicy fragrance use cinnamon, clove, and patchouli; and if you prefer a sweet, floral odor, orange blossom (neroli), jasmine, lavender, and sandalwood will each do the trick. Once you have achieved just the right fragrance, place a bouquet in each room and you will have a magnificent-smelling home.

MINERAL SALT

The tissue, or mineral, salt which is appropriated to Pisces is phosphate of iron (Ferr. Phos.), which is said to oxygenate and purify the blood. This salt helps to maintain normal blood functions, eases respiration, and can help treat sore throats, coughs, colds, fevers, and inflammations. Phosphate of iron strengthens the walls of the blood vessels and arteries, preventing atherosclerosis later in life. A deficiency of this mineral results in anemia or the inability to eliminate toxic waste. Foods rich in phosphate of iron include lettuce, radishes, spinach, dried fruits (dates, raisins, figs, and prunes), beans, strawberries, lentils, onions, cabbage, apples, walnuts, and barley.

GEM AND COLOR THERAPY

If your birthday is between February 19 and February 29, your birthstone is the amethyst, a lovely purple stone which is renowned for its healing ability, especially in the treatment of migraine headaches. If you were born between March 1 and 20, your birthstone is the aquamarine, an exquisite stone which literally means "water" (*aqua*) and "pertaining to the water" (*ma-*

rine), perfectly fitting for the water sign of Pisces. These stones should preferably be set in silver. The color blue has always been utilized for a calming effect and is said to improve relationships by abetting communication. If you cannot make trips to the beach, do the next best thing and keep a blue light shining in your room. Painting the walls blue and wearing shades of blue clothing certainly do not hurt, either.

Chapter 14

Planetary Cycles

———— ✦ ————

A Time for Everything Under the Sun

Once you've assessed the ailments and conditions to which you may be predisposed, the next step entails investigating how the planets' current positions, known as transits, affect your health by increasing or diminishing vitality. From the moment you were born, the planets have been continually traveling through the zodiac according to their individual rate of speed. At different points along its journey, each transiting planet reaches the same zodiacal sign and degree occupied by a planet in your chart, or forms an angle to it. When this happens, the transiting planet lends its influence depending on its particular character traits. (See Table 1.2.) For instance, if Jupiter, the planet of abundance, influences your horoscope, the effect will be one of expansion. Saturn, on the other hand, limits and restricts whatever it touches. With a printout of your chart, you can easily calculate when each transiting planet reaches the degree of, or forms an angle to, a natal planet. If you do not have a copy of your horoscope, you can still weigh the current planetary influences by seeing when they transit your Sun sign (which everyone knows) and the sign of your ascendant (which you can calculate from the tables in Appendix I).

To find out the zodiacal sign and degree (including minutes) of each planet on a given day, the astrologer looks at the ephemeris, his/her most valued tool. The ephemeris, available in book form or as part of an astrological software package (see Appendix V), lists the daily positions of each planet as well as a variety of other astronomical factors of use to the astrologer.

If you do not own astrology software, or an ephemeris, you can refer to Tables 14.1 and 14.2 to view the zodiacal positions for the planets from January 1, 2000, through December 31, 2004. Table 14.1 is a weekly ephemeris which lists the weekly positions of all the planets except for the Moon. To read the table, simply look in the left-hand column for the date you are interested in and read horizontally across for the position of planet in its appropriate column. Each planet is listed according to its degree, sign, and minutes and is calculated for Eastern Standard Time. Since this ephemeris is only calculated at weekly intervals, you will not always be able to ascertain the exact degree and minutes of each planet. It will, however, show you which sign in which the planet is placed as well as its approximate longitude. For example, if you wish to find out where Mars was located on September 11, 2000, you would go to September 9, 2000, and read down the Mars column, where you would find that Mars was located at 26 degrees Leo. (If you wish to discover the exact positions, and do not own software or an ephemeris, see Appendix V for astrological chart services.)

Table 14.2 lists the position of the Moon for every other day from January 1, 2000, through December 31, 2004, and is read the same way you would read Table 14.1. To find the Moon's position on September 11, 2000, you would look in the left-hand column at the date, and then in the next column see that the

Moon is located at 19 degrees Aquarius. Because the Moon travels approximately one degree every two hours and, as a result, enters a new zodiacal sign every two and a half days, it may be more difficult to ascertain the precise degree and sign of the Moon. When in doubt, consult the astrological chart services listed in Appendix V.

Because each planet moves at a different rate of speed, it is easy to see that some planets stay in one sign longer than do others. For instance, the Sun takes about thirty days to travel through one sign, while the Moon takes only two and a half days. It takes Jupiter one year to travel through a zodiacal sign and, therefore, twelve years to travel through the entire zodiac. That means that Jupiter will travel through the sign of your Sun every twelve years, while Saturn, which takes approximately two to two and a half years to travel through one sign and about twenty-nine and a half years to travel through the entire zodiac, will travel through the sign of your Sun every twenty-nine and a half years. Depending on your age, you can easily calculate how many times Jupiter or Saturn has passed through the sign of your Sun or ascendant. If, for instance, you are a Capricorn born in 1953, Jupiter was in the sign of Taurus at the moment of your birth.* Since then, Jupiter has transited the sign of Capricorn, your Sun sign, four times (1960–61, 1972–73, 1984, and 1996–97), while Saturn has passed through the sign of your Sun only twice (1959–60 and 1988–1991). Mars, on the other hand, an indicator of increased energy, fevers, and accidents, takes approximately two years to travel the zodiac and therefore has influenced your Sun and rising signs every other year.

In addition to seeing when each planet passes through your

---

* If you do not own an ephemeris or computer program, Appendix V lists where you can obtain a copy of your birth chart.

Sun and rising signs in the next five years, it is important to take note of the day(s) on which the transits pass over the exact degree of your Sun. If you use Table 14.1, be sure that you estimate the planet's degree on a particular day from its weekly positions. The current planets will exert the following influence when they pass through the sign of your Sun and the sign of your ascendant, both of which you know without obtaining a printout of your chart.

Sun—When the Sun transits through the sign of your Sun or your rising sign for around one month each year, your vitality will increase, and you have the ability to heal yourself once you put your mind to it. There is the feeling that you are the center of the universe and the world is indeed your oyster.

Moon—It takes the Moon two to two and a half days to pass through a zodiacal sign. If that sign is the sign of your Sun or ascendant, you will be more emotional than usual. Take note of any physical complaints which are emotionally related or even psychosomatic, since this is a time they might act up.

Mercury—Mercury's journey through a sign usually lasts about three weeks. Since it is a high-strung, nervous planet, its passage through the sign of your Sun or ascendant will make you restless, talkative, and more nervous than usual. You may have difficulty sleeping so be certain that you drink tranquillizing teas and do relaxation exercises. Curtail your intake of caffeine since it may make you short-tempered.

Venus—Like the Sun, Venus passes through the zodiac in about one year's time. During its transit of your Sun or rising sign, you will be loving, sweet, and generally cooperative. Be careful not to be too indulgent as you may discover you have a sweet tooth, resulting in skin rashes, allergic reactions, and weight gain. If you are prone to hypoglycemia, diabetes, eating disorders, or ailments relating to the skin and kidneys, make sure that you exercise regularly. Venus represents love and friendship, so instead of reaching for something good to eat, call a friend and have some fun.

Mars—It takes Mars about two years to traverse the zodiac. Since this hot planet represents fevers, colds, and inflammations, the message is to slow down and smell the roses. Rather than running around like a chicken without a head, take a deep breath and walk slowly. Take your time and you will avoid bruising, falling, and other physical calamities. Watch your temper. When Mars hits something in your chart, you act before you think, making potential enemies out of long-term friends.

Jupiter—When Jupiter, the planet of expansion and abundance, travels through your Sun or rising sign, you will be energetic, optimistic, and possess the ability to heal yourself. During the year Jupiter traverses your Sun or rising sign, you will experience increased vitality, and you may be keenly aware of new opportunities coming your way. You will be exuberant, enthusiastic, with a desire to acquire healthier habits and begin a physical exercise regime. But be careful. Since Jupiter is the planet of excess and expansion, it is not uncommon to be a little "too" social under Jupiter's influence, and your waistline may expand beyond the place you would like it to go. If you already have a weight problem, be prepared to diet and exercise during Jupiter's transit.

Saturn—Saturn's two-and-a-half-year sojourn through your Sun and rising sign can bring restriction, discipline, and the need to conserve your energy. You may truly feel depressed and more pessimistic than usual. If you generally slip into dark moods and cannot see the brighter side of life, follow the tips laid out throughout this book well in advance of the time when Saturn transits the sensitive points in your chart. Remember that you will probably feel weaker and not as invigorated as usual. Since you need a push to commence physical activity during this time, use ginseng, ginger, garlic, and other stimulating herbs to gather your strength and focus your energy. Do not overdo or tax yourself since you will simply wear yourself out.

Uranus*—During the seven years Uranus travels through the sign of your Sun and rising sign, you might have unexpected aches and pains which will come and go as quickly as your moods. Since Uranus is a quirky planet, you may be more high-strung than usual and your nervous system may be more vulnerable and sensitive than it has in the past. It is vital that you keep your emotions in check, and that you avoid stimulants as much as possible. Ankle sprains and other ligament injuries may occur, especially if you do not look before you leap. As long as you are careful to slow down, and avoid situations in which you have to rush around like a chicken without a head, you should be able to use your accelerated adrenaline levels to your advantage.

Neptune—For the approximately fourteen years it takes Neptune to traverse your Sun sign or rising sign, you may find the ability to concentrate, focus, and achieve discipline extremely difficult to achieve. Neptune's influence is one of confusion, dreaminess, and fatigue and, as a result, attaining your goals may take a little more time than usual during this time. Beginning each day by meditating, or doing simple yoga exercises, allows you to overcome inertia and get down to work

---

* *Because Uranus, Neptune and Pluto travel through the zodiac very slowly, any conditions and ailments caused by these planets will not be constant. Rather, they are general descriptions of conditions which may flare up from time to time.*

without wasting too much time. Eat a balanced diet, exercise regularly, and remember to get plenty of fresh air. This will counteract the tendency to retain water, develop allergies, and discover physical aches and pains for which no immediate cause can be found.

Pluto—Pluto's approximately twelve-year journey through your Sun sign and ascendant can, at times, make you feel as if you are hitting your head against a brick wall. Obstacles seem to constantly get in the way, and you will find yourself discovering untapped resources which you never knew you had. This is a fantastic time for discovering how resilient, courageous, and persevering you really are. With "intensity" being the operative word for any period influenced by Pluto, it is a good time to challenge yourself, take risks, and do anything that is exciting and adventurous but which, until now, seemed intimidating and frightening. If you have ever considered switching professions, returning to school, moving house, working on perfecting your relationships, or making any major changes—internal or external—this is the time to do so. Seek counseling, get involved with community work, or donate time to a charitable organization.

Table 14.1 • Weekly Ephemeris 2000–2005

EST +05:00 Tropical Geo Long	The Sun ☉	Mercury ☿	Venus ♀	Mars ♂	Jupiter ♃	Saturn ♄	Uranus ♅	Neptune ♆	Pluto ♇
Jan 1 2000	10°♑04'	01°♑26'	01°♐12'	27°♒44'	25°♈14'	10°♉24'	14°♒47'	03°♒10'	11°♐26'
Jan 8 2000	17°♑12'	12°♑27'	09°♐41'	03°♓10'	25°♈36'	10°♉18'	15°♒09'	03°♒26'	11°♐40'
Jan 15 2000	24°♑20'	23°♑48'	18°♐13'	08°♓35'	26°♈07'	10°♉17' D	15°♒32'	03°♒41'	11°♐54'
Jan 22 2000	01°♒28'	05°♒33'	26°♐47'	14°♓00'	26°♈47'	10°♉22'	15°♒55'	03°♒57'	12°♐06'
Jan 29 2000	08°♒34'	17°♒40'	05°♑22'	19°♓23'	27°♈35'	10°♉33'	16°♒19'	04°♒13'	12°♐17'
Feb 5 2000	15°♒41'	29°♒46'	13°♑59'	24°♓46'	28°♈31'	10°♉49'	16°♒44'	04°♒29'	12°♐27'
Feb 12 2000	22°♒46'	10°♓29'	22°♑36'	00°♈07'	29°♈34'	11°♉10'	17°♒08'	04°♒45'	12°♐36'
Feb 19 2000	29°♒51'	16°♓43'	01°♒14'	05°♈27'	00°♉43'	11°♉36'	17°♒32'	05°♒00'	12°♐43'
Feb 26 2000	06°♓53'	15°♓24' ℞	09°♒53'	10°♈44'	01°♉57'	12°♉06'	17°♒56'	05°♒14'	12°♐48'
Mar 4 2000	13°♓55'	08°♓39'	18°♒32'	16°♈00'	03°♉17'	12°♉40'	18°♒19'	05°♒28'	12°♐51'
Mar 11 2000	20°♓55'	03°♓28'	27°♒11'	21°♈14'	04°♉41'	13°♉18'	18°♒41'	05°♒40'	12°♐53'
Mar 18 2000	27°♓54'	03°♓19' D	05°♓50'	26°♈25'	06°♉08'	14°♉00'	19°♒02'	05°♒52'	12°♐53' ℞
Mar 25 2000	04°♈51'	07°♓22'	14°♓28'	01°♉34'	07°♉39'	14°♉44'	19°♒22'	06°♒02'	12°♐52'
Apr 1 2000	11°♈46'	14°♓14'	23°♓07'	06°♉41'	09°♉13'	15°♉31'	19°♒40'	06°♒11'	12°♐49'
Apr 8 2000	18°♈40'	23°♓03'	01°♈46'	11°♉46'	10°♉49'	16°♉20'	19°♒56'	06°♒19'	12°♐44'
Apr 15 2000	25°♈32'	03°♈23'	10°♈24'	16°♉48'	12°♉26'	17°♉11'	20°♒10'	06°♒25'	12°♐38'
Apr 22 2000	02°♉22'	15°♈04'	19°♈01'	21°♉48'	14°♉05'	18°♉03'	20°♒22'	06°♒30'	12°♐31'
Apr 29 2000	09°♉11'	28°♈07'	27°♈38'	26°♉45'	15°♉44'	18°♉56'	20°♒32'	06°♒32'	12°♐22'
May 6 2000	15°♉58'	12°♉28'	06°♉16'	01°♊41'	17°♉24'	19°♉50'	20°♒40'	06°♒34'	12°♐13'
May 13 2000	22°♉44'	27°♉38'	14°♉52'	06°♊34'	19°♉04'	20°♉44'	20°♒45'	06°♒34' ℞	12°♐03'
May 20 2000	29°♉29'	12°♊19'	23°♉29'	11°♊24'	20°♉44'	21°♉38'	20°♒48'	06°♒32'	11°♐52'
May 27 2000	06°♊12'	25°♊13'	02°♊05'	16°♊13'	22°♉22'	22°♉32'	20°♒49' ℞	06°♒28'	11°♐41'
Jun 3 2000	12°♊55'	05°♋44'	10°♊41'	21°♊00'	24°♉00'	23°♉24'	20°♒47'	06°♒23'	11°♐29'
Jun 10 2000	19°♊37'	13°♋37'	19°♊17'	25°♊44'	25°♉36'	24°♉16'	20°♒43'	06°♒17'	11°♐18'
Jun 17 2000	26°♊18'	18°♋31'	27°♊53'	00°♋27'	27°♉10'	25°♉06'	20°♒36'	06°♒10'	11°♐07'
Jun 24 2000	02°♋59'	19°♋56' ℞	06°♋29'	05°♋08'	28°♉42'	25°♉54'	20°♒28'	06°♒01'	10°♐56'
Jul 1 2000	09°♋39'	17°♋47'	15°♋05'	09°♋47'	00°♊11'	26°♉39'	20°♒18'	05°♒52'	10°♐46'
Jul 8 2000	16°♋20'	13°♋38'	23°♋41'	14°♋25'	01°♊36'	27°♉22'	20°♒05'	05°♒42'	10°♐37'
Jul 15 2000	23°♋00'	10°♋37'	02°♌18'	19°♋01'	02°♊58'	28°♉03'	19°♒52'	05°♒31'	10°♐29'
Jul 22 2000	29°♋41'	11°♋23' D	10°♌54'	23°♋35'	04°♊16'	28°♉39'	19°♒37'	05°♒20'	10°♐22'
Jul 29 2000	06°♌22'	16°♋47'	19°♌31'	28°♋09'	05°♊29'	29°♉13'	19°♒21'	05°♒08'	10°♐17'
Aug 5 2000	13°♌04'	26°♋30'	28°♌07'	02°♌41'	06°♊36'	29°♉42'	19°♒05'	04°♒57'	10°♐12'
Aug 12 2000	19°♌47'	09°♌24'	06°♍44'	07°♌11'	07°♊38'	00°♊07'	18°♒48'	04°♒46'	10°♐10'
Aug 19 2000	26°♌23'	23°♌33'	15°♍20'	11°♌41'	08°♊33'	00°♊27'	18°♒31'	04°♒35'	10°♐09'
Aug 26 2000	03°♍15'	07°♍22'	23°♍56'	16°♌09'	09°♊21'	00°♊42'	18°♒15'	04°♒25'	10°♐09' D
Sep 2 2000	10°♍01'	20°♍14'	02°♎31'	20°♌37'	10°♊01'	00°♊53'	17°♒59'	04°♒16'	10°♐11'
Sep 9 2000	16°♍49'	02°♎05'	11°♎06'	25°♌03'	10°♊33'	00°♊58'	17°♒45'	04°♒08'	10°♐15'
Sep 16 2000	23°♍37'	13°♎00'	19°♎41'	29°♌29'	10°♊56'	00°♊57' ℞	17°♒32'	04°♒01'	10°♐20'
Sep 23 2000	00°♎28'	23°♎01'	28°♎14'	03°♍54'	11°♊10'	00°♊52'	17°♒20'	03°♒55'	10°♐27'
Sep 30 2000	07°♎20'	02°♏00'	06°♏47'	08°♍18'	11°♊14' ℞	00°♊41'	17°♒10'	03°♒51'	10°♐35'
Oct 7 2000	14°♎14'	09°♏34'	15°♏20'	12°♍41'	11°♊08'	00°♊26'	17°♒03'	03°♒48'	10°♐45'
Oct 14 2000	21°♎09'	14°♏42'	23°♏51'	17°♍03'	10°♊52'	00°♊06'	16°♒57'	03°♒47'	10°♐56'
Oct 21 2000	28°♎06'	15°♏19' ℞	02°♐21'	21°♍24'	10°♊27'	29°♉41'	16°♒54'	03°♒47' D	11°♐08'
Oct 28 2000	05°♏04'	09°♏21'	10°♐50'	25°♍45'	09°♊53'	29°♉13'	16°♒53' D	03°♒50'	11°♐21'
Nov 4 2000	12°♏05'	01°♏23'	19°♐18'	00°♎04'	09°♊11'	28°♉42'	16°♒55'	03°♒53'	11°♐35'
Nov 11 2000	19°♏06'	00°♏47' D	27°♐44'	04°♎22'	08°♊22'	28°♉09'	16°♒59'	03°♒59'	11°♐50'
Nov 18 2000	26°♏09'	07°♏18'	06°♑07'	08°♎40'	07°♊29'	27°♉35'	17°♒06'	04°♒06'	12°♐06'
Nov 25 2000	03°♐13'	16°♏54'	14°♑28'	12°♎58'	06°♊32'	27°♉01'	17°♒15'	04°♒14'	12°♐22'
Dec 2 2000	10°♐19'	27°♏28'	22°♑45'	17°♎11'	05°♊35'	26°♉28'	17°♒27'	04°♒24'	12°♐38'
Dec 9 2000	17°♐25'	08°♐17'	00°♒59'	21°♎24'	04°♊39'	25°♉56'	17°♒41'	04°♒35'	12°♐54'
Dec 16 2000	24°♐32'	19°♐11'	09°♒06'	25°♎36'	03°♊47'	25°♉27'	17°♒56'	04°♒48'	13°♐10'
Dec 23 2000	01°♑40'	00°♑11'	17°♒06'	29°♎45'	03°♊00'	25°♉01'	18°♒14'	05°♒01'	13°♐26'
Dec 30 2000	08°♑48'	11°♑22'	24°♒58'	03°♏53'	02°♊20'	24°♉40'	18°♒33'	05°♒15'	13°♐42'
Jan 6 2001	15°♑56'	22°♑47'	02°♓39'	07°♏58'	01°♊48'	24°♉23'	18°♒54'	05°♒30'	13°♐56'
Jan 13 2001	23°♑04'	04°♒24'	10°♓06'	12°♏00'	01°♊26'	24°♉11'	19°♒16'	05°♒46'	14°♐10'
Jan 20 2001	00°♒12'	15°♒49'	17°♓15'	15°♏59'	01°♊13'	24°♉04'	19°♒39'	06°♒02'	14°♐23'
Jan 27 2001	07°♒19'	25°♒39'	24°♓02'	19°♏55'	01°♊11' D	24°♉03' D	20°♒02'	06°♒17'	14°♐35'
Feb 3 2001	14°♒25'	02°♓37'	00°♈21'	23°♏46'	01°♊19'	24°♉08'	20°♒27'	06°♒33'	14°♐45'
Feb 10 2001	21°♒31'	27°♒25' ℞	06°♈01'	27°♏33'	01°♊36'	24°♉18'	20°♒51'	06°♒49'	14°♐54'
Feb 17 2001	28°♒35'	19°♒40'	10°♈52'	01°♐14'	02°♊03'	24°♉33'	21°♒15'	07°♒04'	15°♐02'
Feb 24 2001	05°♓38'	15°♒31'	14°♈39'	04°♐48'	02°♊39'	24°♉54'	21°♒39'	07°♒19'	15°♐08'
Mar 3 2001	12°♓40'	16°♒57' D	17°♈03'	08°♐16'	03°♊23'	25°♉19'	22°♒03'	07°♒33'	15°♐12'
Mar 10 2001	19°♓41'	22°♒15'	17°♈42' ℞	11°♐34'	04°♊14'	25°♉49'	22°♒26'	07°♒46'	15°♐15'

EST +05:00 Tropical Geo Long	The Sun ☉	Mercury ☿	Venus ♀	Mars ♂	Jupiter ♃	Saturn ♄	Uranus ♅	Neptune ♆	Pluto ♇
Mar 17 2001	26°♓39'	29°♒56'	16°♈21'	14°♐43'	05°♊13'	26°♉23'	22°♒47'	07°♒59'	15°♐16'
Mar 24 2001	03°♈37'	09°♓15'	13°♈09'	17°♐40'	06°♊18'	27°♉01'	23°♒08'	08°♒10'	15°♐15' ℞
Mar 31 2001	10°♈32'	19°♓50'	08°♈52'	20°♐22'	07°♊28'	27°♉42'	23°♒27'	08°♒19'	15°♐13'
Apr 7 2001	17°♈26'	01°♈35'	04°♈49'	22°♐49'	08°♊43'	28°♉26'	23°♒45'	08°♒28'	15°♐09'
Apr 14 2001	24°♈18'	14°♈32'	02°♈10'	24°♐56'	10°♊03'	29°♉13'	24°♒00'	08°♒34'	15°♐04'
Apr 21 2001	01°♉09'	28°♈40'	01°♈28' D	26°♐41'	11°♊27'	00°♊02'	24°♒14'	08°♒40'	14°♐58'
Apr 28 2001	07°♉58'	13°♉35'	02°♈39'	27°♐59'	12°♊54'	00°♊52'	24°♒26'	08°♒43'	14°♐50'
May 5 2001	14°♉46'	28°♉04'	05°♈23'	28°♐47'	14°♊23'	01°♊45'	24°♒35'	08°♒46'	14°♐41'
May 12 2001	21°♉32'	10°♊35'	09°♈22'	29°♐02' ℞	15°♊55'	02°♊38'	24°♒42'	08°♒46' ℞	14°♐31'
May 19 2001	28°♉17'	20°♊18'	14°♈17'	28°♐41'	17°♊29'	03°♊32'	24°♒47'	08°♒45'	14°♐21'
May 26 2001	05°♊01'	26°♊50'	19°♈54'	27°♐42'	19°♊04'	04°♊26'	24°♒49'	08°♒42'	14°♐10'
Jun 2 2001	11°♊43'	29°♊48'	26°♈04'	26°♐10'	20°♊40'	05°♊21'	24°♒49' ℞	08°♒38'	13°♐58'
Jun 9 2001	18°♊25'	29°♊04' ℞	02°♉39'	24°♐11'	22°♊17'	06°♊15'	24°♒47'	08°♒33'	13°♐47'
Jun 16 2001	25°♊07'	25°♊39'	09°♉33'	21°♐57'	23°♊54'	07°♊08'	24°♒42'	08°♒26'	13°♐36'
Jun 23 2001	01°♋48'	22°♊11'	16°♉43'	19°♐43'	25°♊30'	08°♊00'	24°♒35'	08°♒18'	13°♐25'
Jun 30 2001	08°♋28'	21°♊25' D	24°♉05'	17°♐44'	27°♊07'	08°♊51'	24°♒27'	08°♒09'	13°♐15'
Jul 7 2001	15°♋09'	24°♊31'	01°♊38'	16°♐14'	28°♊42'	09°♊39'	24°♒16'	07°♒59'	13°♐05'
Jul 14 2001	21°♋49'	01°♋32'	09°♊20'	15°♐20'	00°♋16'	10°♊26'	24°♒03'	07°♒48'	12°♐57'
Jul 21 2001	28°♋30'	12°♋05'	17°♊09'	15°♐07' D	01°♋48'	11°♊10'	23°♒49'	07°♒37'	12°♐49'
Jul 28 2001	05°♌11'	25°♋25'	25°♊04'	15°♐35'	03°♋18'	11°♊51'	23°♒34'	07°♒26'	12°♐43'
Aug 4 2001	11°♌53'	09°♌59'	03°♋05'	16°♐42'	04°♋45'	12°♊29'	23°♒18'	07°♒15'	12°♐38'
Aug 11 2001	18°♌36'	24°♌12'	11°♋12'	18°♐23'	06°♋09'	13°♊04'	23°♒02'	07°♒03'	12°♐34'
Aug 18 2001	25°♌19'	07°♍22'	19°♋24'	20°♐36'	07°♋30'	13°♊34'	22°♒45'	06°♒53'	12°♐32'
Aug 25 2001	02°♍04'	19°♍22'	27°♋39'	23°♐16'	08°♋46'	14°♊00'	22°♒28'	06°♒42'	12°♐32' D
Sep 1 2001	08°♍49'	00°♎16'	05°♌59'	26°♐20'	09°♋58'	14°♊22'	22°♒12'	06°♒33'	12°♐33'
Sep 8 2001	15°♍36'	10°♎03'	14°♌23'	29°♐43'	11°♋05'	14°♊38'	21°♒57'	06°♒24'	12°♐36'
Sep 15 2001	22°♍25'	18°♎35'	22°♌51'	03°♑24'	12°♋06'	14°♊50'	21°♒42'	06°♒16'	12°♐40'
Sep 22 2001	29°♍15'	25°♎22'	01°♍21'	07°♑20'	13°♋01'	14°♊56'	21°♒30'	06°♒10'	12°♐46'
Sep 29 2001	06°♎07'	29°♎18'	09°♍55'	11°♑29'	13°♋48'	14°♊57' ℞	21°♒18'	06°♒05'	12°♐54'
Oct 6 2001	13°♎00'	28°♎29' ℞	18°♍31'	15°♑49'	14°♋28'	14°♊53'	21°♒09'	06°♒01'	13°♐02'
Oct 13 2001	19°♎55'	21°♎49'	27°♍10'	20°♑18'	15°♋00'	14°♊43'	21°♒02'	05°♒59'	13°♐13'
Oct 20 2001	26°♎52'	14°♎56'	05°♎51'	24°♑55'	15°♋23'	14°♊29'	20°♒57'	05°♒59' D	13°♐24'
Oct 27 2001	03°♏50'	15°♎44' D	14°♎34'	29°♑38'	15°♋37'	14°♊09'	20°♒54'	06°♒00'	13°♐37'
Nov 3 2001	10°♏50'	23°♎17'	23°♎18'	04°♒28'	15°♋41' ℞	13°♊45'	20°♒54' D	06°♒03'	13°♐51'
Nov 10 2001	17°♏51'	03°♏40'	02°♏03'	09°♒22'	15°♋35'	13°♊18'	20°♒57'	06°♒08'	14°♐05'
Nov 17 2001	24°♏54'	14°♏47'	10°♏50'	14°♒19'	15°♋20'	12°♊47'	21°♒02'	06°♒14'	14°♐20'
Nov 24 2001	01°♐58'	25°♏56'	19°♏37'	19°♒20'	14°♋55'	12°♊14'	21°♒09'	06°♒22'	14°♐36'
Dec 1 2001	09°♐03'	07°♐00'	28°♏25'	24°♒24'	14°♋21'	11°♊40'	21°♒19'	06°♒31'	14°♐52'
Dec 8 2001	16°♐09'	18°♐00'	07°♐13'	29°♒29'	13°♋39'	11°♊06'	21°♒31'	06°♒42'	15°♐08'
Dec 15 2001	23°♐16'	29°♐01'	16°♐01'	04°♓35'	12°♋51'	10°♊32'	21°♒45'	06°♒54'	15°♐24'
Dec 22 2001	00°♑24'	10°♑06'	24°♐50'	09°♓42'	11°♋58'	10°♊00'	22°♒01'	07°♒07'	15°♐40'
Dec 29 2001	07°♑32'	21°♑13'	03°♑38'	14°♓50'	11°♋02'	09°♊30'	22°♒19'	07°♒20'	15°♐56'
Jan 5 2002	14°♑40'	01°♒55'	12°♑27'	19°♓57'	10°♋05'	09°♊04'	22°♒39'	07°♒35'	16°♐11'
Jan 12 2002	21°♑48'	10°♒48'	21°♑15'	25°♓04'	09°♋10'	08°♊41'	23°♒00'	07°♒50'	16°♐25'
Jan 19 2002	28°♑56'	14°♒28' ℞	00°♒04'	00°♈11'	08°♋18'	08°♊23'	23°♒22'	08°♒06'	16°♐38'
Jan 26 2002	06°♒03'	09°♒36'	08°♒51'	05°♈16'	07°♋31'	08°♊11'	23°♒45'	08°♒22'	16°♐50'
Feb 2 2002	13°♒09'	01°♒29'	17°♒39'	10°♈21'	06°♋50'	08°♊03'	24°♒09'	08°♒38'	17°♐01'
Feb 9 2002	20°♒15'	28°♑38' D	26°♒26'	15°♈24'	06°♋18'	08°♊01' D	24°♒33'	08°♒54'	17°♐11'
Feb 16 2002	27°♒20'	01°♒31'	05°♓12'	20°♈25'	05°♋55'	08°♊05'	24°♒57'	09°♒09'	17°♐19'
Feb 23 2002	04°♓23'	07°♒51'	13°♓57'	25°♈26'	05°♋41'	08°♊14'	25°♒22'	09°♒24'	17°♐26'
Mar 2 2002	11°♓25'	16°♒11'	22°♓41'	00°♉24'	05°♋37' D	08°♊29'	25°♒45'	09°♒39'	17°♐31'
Mar 9 2002	18°♓26'	25°♒52'	01°♈24'	05°♉21'	05°♋43'	08°♊49'	26°♒09'	09°♒52'	17°♐35'
Mar 16 2002	25°♓25'	06°♓36'	10°♈07'	10°♉16'	05°♋58'	09°♊13'	26°♒31'	10°♒05'	17°♐37'
Mar 23 2002	02°♈23'	18°♓20'	18°♈47'	15°♉09'	06°♋22'	09°♊42'	26°♒53'	10°♒16'	17°♐37' ℞
Mar 30 2002	09°♈18'	01°♈07'	27°♈26'	20°♉01'	06°♋55'	10°♊16'	27°♒13'	10°♒27'	17°♐36'
Apr 6 2002	16°♈13'	14°♈58'	06°♉04'	24°♉50'	07°♋35'	10°♊53'	27°♒31'	10°♒36'	17°♐33'
Apr 13 2002	23°♈05'	29°♈32'	14°♉40'	29°♉38'	08°♋24'	11°♊34'	27°♒48'	10°♒43'	17°♐28'
Apr 20 2002	29°♈56'	13°♉42'	23°♉14'	04°♊24'	09°♋19'	12°♊17'	28°♒04'	10°♒49'	17°♐22'
Apr 27 2002	06°♉45'	25°♉43'	01°♊46'	09°♊08'	10°♋20'	13°♊04'	28°♒17'	10°♒54'	17°♐15'
May 4 2002	13°♉33'	04°♊22'	10°♊16'	13°♊51'	11°♋26'	13°♊52'	28°♒28'	10°♒57'	17°♐07'
May 11 2002	20°♉20'	09°♊07'	18°♊44'	18°♊32'	12°♋38'	14°♊43'	28°♒37'	10°♒58'	16°♐57'
May 18 2002	27°♉05'	09°♊45' ℞	27°♊10'	23°♊12'	13°♋54'	15°♊35'	28°♒44'	10°♒58' ℞	16°♐47'
May 25 2002	03°♊49'	06°♊59'	05°♋33'	27°♊50'	15°♋13'	16°♊28'	28°♒48'	10°♒56'	16°♐37'

EST +05:00 Tropical Geo Long	The Sun ☉	Mercury ☿	Venus ♀	Mars ♂	Jupiter ♃	Saturn ♄	Uranus ♅	Neptune ♆	Pluto ♇
Jun 1 2002	10°♊32'	03°♊12'	13°♋54'	02°♋26'	16°♋36'	17°♊22'	28°♒50'	10°♒53'	16°♐26'
Jun 8 2002	17°♊14'	01°♊21'	22°♋11'	07°♋02'	18°♋02'	18°♊17'	28°♒49' ℞	10°♒48'	16°♐14'
Jun 15 2002	23°♊56'	02°♊58' D	00°♌25'	11°♋36'	19°♋31'	19°♊12'	28°♒46'	10°♒42'	16°♐03'
Jun 22 2002	00°♋37'	08°♊08'	08°♌35'	16°♋09'	21°♋01'	20°♊06'	28°♒41'	10°♒34'	15°♐52'
Jun 29 2002	07°♋17'	16°♊29'	16°♌41'	20°♋41'	22°♋32'	20°♊59'	28°♒33'	10°♒26'	15°♐42'
Jul 6 2002	13°♋58'	27°♊44'	24°♌42'	25°♋12'	24°♋05'	21°♊52'	28°♒24'	10°♒16'	15°♐32'
Jul 13 2002	20°♋38'	11°♋25'	02°♍37'	29°♋43'	25°♋39'	22°♊43'	28°♒13'	10°♒06'	15°♐23'
Jul 20 2002	27°♋19'	26°♋18'	10°♍25'	04°♌12'	27°♋12'	23°♊33'	28°♒00'	09°♒55'	15°♐15'
Jul 27 2002	04°♌00'	10°♌52'	18°♍05'	08°♌41'	28°♋46'	24°♊20'	27°♒46'	09°♒44'	15°♐08'
Aug 3 2002	10°♌42'	24°♌17'	25°♍36'	13°♌10'	00°♌19'	25°♊05'	27°♒30'	09°♒33'	15°♐02'
Aug 10 2002	17°♌24'	06°♍24'	02°♎56'	17°♌38'	01°♌52'	25°♊48'	27°♒14'	09°♒21'	14°♐58'
Aug 17 2002	24°♌08'	17°♍14'	10°♎01'	22°♌06'	03°♌23'	26°♊27'	26°♒58'	09°♒10'	14°♐55'
Aug 24 2002	00°♍52'	26°♍45'	16°♎49'	26°♌33'	04°♌52'	27°♊02'	26°♒41'	08°♒59'	14°♐53'
Aug 31 2002	07°♍37'	04°♎43'	23°♎16'	01°♍01'	06°♌20'	27°♊34'	26°♒24'	08°♒49'	14°♐54' D
Sep 7 2002	14°♍24'	10°♎36'	29°♎15'	05°♍28'	07°♌44'	28°♊01'	26°♒08'	08°♒40'	14°♐56'
Sep 14 2002	21°♍13'	13°♎13'	04°♏38'	09°♍55'	09°♌06'	28°♊24'	25°♒53'	08°♒32'	14°♐59'
Sep 21 2002	28°♍02'	10°♎57' ℞	09°♏14'	14°♍22'	10°♌24'	28°♊42'	25°♒39'	08°♒25'	15°♐04'
Sep 28 2002	04°♎54'	03°♎59'	12°♏48'	18°♍49'	11°♌39'	28°♊55'	25°♒27'	08°♒19'	15°♐11'
Oct 5 2002	11°♎47'	28°♍32'	15°♏01'	23°♍17'	12°♌48'	29°♊02'	25°♒16'	08°♒15'	15°♐19'
Oct 12 2002	18°♎42'	00°♎46' D	15°♏34' ℞	27°♍45'	13°♌52'	29°♊05' ℞	25°♒07'	08°♒12'	15°♐29'
Oct 19 2002	25°♎38'	09°♎18'	14°♏11'	02°♎12'	14°♌51'	29°♊01'	25°♒00'	08°♒11'	15°♐39'
Oct 26 2002	02°♏36'	20°♎26'	11°♏00'	06°♎41'	15°♌43'	28°♊53'	24°♒56'	08°♒12' D	15°♐51'
Nov 2 2002	09°♏35'	02°♏05'	06°♏51'	11°♎09'	16°♌27'	28°♊39'	24°♒54'	08°♒14'	16°♐04'
Nov 9 2002	16°♏37'	13°♏36'	03°♏00'	15°♎38'	17°♌05'	28°♊20'	24°♒55' D	08°♒18'	16°♐18'
Nov 16 2002	23°♏39'	24°♏50'	00°♏35'	20°♎07'	17°♌33'	27°♊57'	24°♒58'	08°♒23'	16°♐33'
Nov 23 2002	00°♐43'	05°♐50'	00°♏07' D	24°♎36'	17°♌53'	27°♊30'	25°♒03'	08°♒30'	16°♐48'
Nov 30 2002	07°♐48'	16°♐42'	01°♏35'	29°♎06'	18°♌04'	27°♊00'	25°♒11'	08°♒39'	17°♐04'
Dec 7 2002	14°♐54'	27°♐29'	04°♏38'	03°♏36'	18°♌05' ℞	26°♊27'	25°♒22'	08°♒49'	17°♐20'
Dec 14 2002	22°♐01'	08°♑05'	08°♏56'	08°♏06'	17°♌56'	25°♊53'	25°♒34'	09°♒00'	17°♐36'
Dec 21 2002	29°♐08'	18°♑03'	14°♏12'	12°♏36'	17°♌38'	25°♊18'	25°♒49'	09°♒12'	17°♐52'
Dec 28 2002	06°♑16'	25°♑55'	20°♏11'	17°♏07'	17°♌11'	24°♊44'	26°♒05'	09°♒26'	18°♐08'
Jan 4 2003	13°♑24'	28°♑15' ℞	26°♏43'	21°♏38'	16°♌36'	24°♊11'	26°♒24'	09°♒40'	18°♐23'
Jan 11 2003	20°♑32'	22°♑00'	03°♐41'	26°♏08'	15°♌53'	23°♊41'	26°♒44'	09°♒55'	18°♐38'
Jan 18 2003	27°♑40'	14°♑01'	10°♐57'	00°♐39'	15°♌04'	23°♊14'	27°♒05'	10°♒10'	18°♐51'
Jan 25 2003	04°♒47'	12°♑35' D	18°♐30'	05°♐10'	14°♌11'	22°♊51'	27°♒27'	10°♒26'	19°♐04'
Feb 1 2003	11°♒54'	16°♑47'	26°♐14'	09°♐41'	13°♌15'	22°♊32'	27°♒51'	10°♒42'	19°♐16'
Feb 8 2003	19°♒00'	24°♑00'	04°♑07'	14°♐11'	12°♌19'	22°♊19'	28°♒14'	10°♒58'	19°♐26'
Feb 15 2003	26°♒05'	02°♒52'	12°♑08'	18°♐41'	11°♌25'	22°♊10'	28°♒39'	11°♒14'	19°♐35'
Feb 22 2003	03°♓08'	12°♒49'	20°♑15'	23°♐10'	10°♌35'	22°♊08'	29°♒03'	11°♒29'	19°♐42'
Mar 1 2003	10°♓11'	23°♒38'	28°♑26'	27°♐39'	09°♌50'	22°♊10' D	29°♒27'	11°♒44'	19°♐48'
Mar 8 2003	17°♓12'	05°♓18'	06°♒42'	02°♑06'	09°♌11'	22°♊18'	29°♒51'	11°♒58'	19°♐53'
Mar 15 2003	24°♓11'	17°♓53'	15°♒00'	06°♑33'	08°♌41'	22°♊32'	00°♓14'	12°♒11'	19°♐55'
Mar 22 2003	01°♈09'	01°♈23'	23°♒21'	10°♑58'	08°♌19'	22°♊51'	00°♓36'	12°♒23'	19°♐56'
Mar 29 2003	08°♈05'	15°♈32'	01°♓44'	15°♑22'	08°♌07'	23°♊14'	00°♓57'	12°♒34'	19°♐56' ℞
Apr 5 2003	15°♈00'	29°♈15'	10°♓08'	19°♑44'	08°♌03' D	23°♊43'	01°♓17'	12°♒44'	19°♐54'
Apr 12 2003	21°♈53'	10°♉37'	18°♓34'	24°♑03'	08°♌09'	24°♊15'	01°♓35'	12°♒52'	19°♐50'
Apr 19 2003	28°♈44'	17°♉58'	27°♓00'	28°♑19'	08°♌24'	24°♊52'	01°♓52'	12°♒59'	19°♐45'
Apr 26 2003	05°♉33'	20°♉32'	05°♈28'	02°♒31'	08°♌48'	25°♊31'	02°♓06'	13°♒04'	19°♐38'
May 3 2003	12°♉22'	18°♉42' ℞	13°♈56'	06°♒39'	09°♌20'	26°♊14'	02°♓19'	13°♒08'	19°♐30'
May 10 2003	19°♉08'	14°♉33'	22°♈25'	10°♒42'	10°♌00'	27°♊00'	02°♓30'	13°♒10'	19°♐22'
May 17 2003	25°♉54'	11°♉29'	00°♉54'	14°♒37'	10°♌47'	27°♊48'	02°♓38'	13°♒11' ℞	19°♐12'
May 24 2003	02°♊38'	11°♉41' D	09°♉24'	18°♒26'	11°♌40'	28°♊39'	02°♓44'	13°♒10'	19°♐02'
May 31 2003	09°♊21'	15°♉28'	17°♉54'	22°♒04'	12°♌39'	29°♊30'	02°♓47'	13°♒07'	18°♐51'
Jun 7 2003	16°♊03'	22°♉17'	26°♉25'	25°♒31'	13°♌44'	00°♋23'	02°♓49' ℞	13°♒03'	18°♐40'
Jun 14 2003	22°♊45'	01°♊42'	04°♊56'	28°♒44'	14°♌53'	01°♋17'	02°♓48'	12°♒57'	18°♐29'
Jun 21 2003	29°♊26'	13°♊30'	13°♊28'	01°♓41'	16°♌07'	02°♋12'	02°♓44'	12°♒51'	18°♐18'
Jun 28 2003	06°♋06'	27°♊24'	22°♊01'	04°♓17'	17°♌24'	03°♋06'	02°♓38'	12°♒43'	18°♐07'
Jul 5 2003	12°♋47'	12°♋31'	00°♋34'	06°♓30'	18°♌45'	04°♋01'	02°♓31'	12°♒33'	17°♐57'
Jul 12 2003	19°♋27'	27°♋21'	09°♋08'	08°♓14'	20°♌08'	04°♋55'	02°♓21'	12°♒24'	17°♐47'
Jul 19 2003	26°♋08'	10°♌59'	17°♋44'	09°♓27'	21°♌34'	05°♋48'	02°♓09'	12°♒13'	17°♐39'
Jul 26 2003	02°♌49'	23°♌08'	26°♋20'	10°♓04'	23°♌02'	06°♋40'	01°♓56'	12°♒02'	17°♐31'
Aug 2 2003	09°♌31'	03°♍49'	04°♌57'	10°♓01' ℞	24°♌31'	07°♋30'	01°♓41'	11°♒51'	17°♐25'
Aug 9 2003	16°♌13'	12°♍57'	13°♌35'	09°♓21'	26°♌02'	08°♋18'	01°♓26'	11°♒39'	17°♐20'

EST +05:00 Tropical Geo Long	The Sun ☉	Mercury ☿	Venus ♀	Mars ♂	Jupiter ♃	Saturn ♄	Uranus ♅	Neptune ♆	Pluto ♇
Aug 16 2003	22°♌56'	20°♍15'	22°♌14'	08°♓08'	27°♌33'	09°♋04'	01°♓09'	11°♒28'	17°♐16'
Aug 23 2003	29°♌40'	25°♍02'	00°♍53'	06°♓29'	29°♌05'	09°♋47'	00°♓53'	11°♒17'	17°♐14'
Aug 30 2003	06°♍25'	26°♍11' ℞	09°♍34'	04°♓37'	00°♍36'	10°♋27'	00°♓36'	11°♒07'	17°♐13' D
Sep 6 2003	13°♍12'	22°♍35'	18°♍15'	02°♓51'	02°♍07'	11°♋03'	00°♓20'	10°♒57'	17°♐15'
Sep 13 2003	20°♍00'	15°♍53'	26°♍56'	01°♓24'	03°♍38'	11°♋36'	00°♓04'	10°♒48'	17°♐17'
Sep 20 2003	26°♍49'	12°♍12'	05°♎38'	00°♓27'	05°♍06'	12°♋04'	29°♒49'	10°♒41'	17°♐21'
Sep 27 2003	03°♎41'	15°♍51' D	14°♎21'	00°♓07'	06°♍34'	12°♋28'	29°♒35'	10°♒34'	17°♐27'
Oct 4 2003	10°♎33'	25°♍18'	23°♎03'	00°♓26' D	07°♍59'	12°♋48'	29°♒23'	10°♒29'	17°♐35'
Oct 11 2003	17°♎28'	07°♎09'	01°♏45'	01°♓23'	09°♍21'	13°♋02'	29°♒13'	10°♒26'	17°♐43'
Oct 18 2003	24°♎24'	19°♎21'	10°♏28'	02°♓54'	10°♍40'	13°♋10'	29°♒04'	10°♒24'	17°♐53'
Oct 25 2003	01°♏21'	01°♏13'	19°♏10'	04°♓55'	11°♍55'	13°♋14'	28°♒58'	10°♒24' D	18°♐05'
Nov 1 2003	08°♏21'	12°♏38'	27°♏53'	07°♓23'	13°♍06'	13°♋12' ℞	28°♒55'	10°♒25'	18°♐17'
Nov 8 2003	15°♏22'	23°♏41'	06°♐35'	10°♓13'	14°♍13'	13°♋04'	28°♒53'	10°♒28'	18°♐31'
Nov 15 2003	22°♏24'	04°♐25'	15°♐17'	13°♓21'	15°♍13'	12°♋51'	28°♒54' D	10°♒33'	18°♐45'
Nov 22 2003	29°♏27'	14°♐53'	23°♐59'	16°♓44'	16°♍08'	12°♋33'	28°♒58'	10°♒39'	19°♐00'
Nov 29 2003	06°♐32'	24°♐58'	02°♑40'	20°♓21'	16°♍56'	12°♋11'	29°♒04'	10°♒47'	19°♐15'
Dec 6 2003	13°♐38'	04°♑10'	11°♑21'	24°♓08'	17°♍36'	11°♋44'	29°♒13'	10°♒56'	19°♐31'
Dec 13 2003	20°♐45'	10°♑58'	20°♑01'	28°♓04'	18°♍09'	11°♋15'	29°♒24'	11°♒07'	19°♐47'
Dec 20 2003	27°♐52'	11°♑57' ℞	28°♑41'	02°♈07'	18°♍33'	10°♋42'	29°♒37'	11°♒18'	20°♐03'
Dec 27 2003	05°♑00'	04°♑37'	07°♒19'	06°♈16'	18°♍48'	10°♋08'	29°♒52'	11°♒31'	20°♐19'
Jan 3 2004	12°♑08'	27°♐10'	15°♒55'	10°♈30'	18°♍54'	09°♋34'	00°♓09'	11°♒45'	20°♐34'
Jan 10 2004	19°♑16'	27°♐09' D	24°♒29'	14°♈48'	18°♍50' ℞	08°♋59'	00°♓28'	12°♒00'	20°♐49'
Jan 17 2004	26°♑24'	02°♑32'	03°♓01'	19°♈09'	18°♍37'	08°♋26'	00°♓48'	12°♒15'	21°♐03'
Jan 24 2004	03°♒31'	10°♑32'	11°♓30'	23°♈32'	18°♍15'	07°♋56'	01°♓10'	12°♒31'	21°♐16'
Jan 31 2004	10°♒38'	19°♑52'	19°♓55'	27°♈57'	17°♍44'	07°♋28'	01°♓32'	12°♒47'	21°♐28'
Feb 7 2004	17°♒44'	00°♒02'	28°♓15'	02°♉24'	17°♍05'	07°♋04'	01°♓56'	13°♒03'	21°♐39'
Feb 14 2004	24°♒49'	10°♒54'	06°♈30'	06°♉52'	16°♍20'	06°♋45'	02°♓19'	13°♒18'	21°♐48'
Feb 21 2004	01°♓53'	22°♒28'	14°♈38'	11°♉20'	15°♍30'	06°♋30'	02°♓44'	13°♒34'	21°♐57'
Feb 28 2004	08°♓56'	04°♓47'	22°♈38'	15°♉49'	14°♍36'	06°♋21'	03°♓08'	13°♒49'	22°♐03'
Mar 6 2004	15°♓57'	17°♓54'	00°♉29'	20°♉18'	13°♍42'	06°♋17'	03°♓32'	14°♒03'	22°♐08'
Mar 13 2004	22°♓57'	01°♈34'	08°♉09'	24°♉48'	12°♍47'	06°♋18' D	03°♓55'	14°♒17'	22°♐12'
Mar 20 2004	29°♓55'	14°♈45'	15°♉36'	29°♉17'	11°♍55'	06°♋25'	04°♓18'	14°♒30'	22°♐14'
Mar 27 2004	06°♈52'	25°♈21'	22°♉46'	03°♊46'	11°♍08'	06°♋38'	04°♓40'	14°♒41'	22°♐14' ℞
Apr 3 2004	13°♈46'	01°♉09'	29°♉36'	08°♊15'	10°♍26'	06°♋55'	05°♓01'	14°♒52'	22°♐13'
Apr 10 2004	20°♈39'	01°♉19' ℞	06°♊00'	12°♊43'	09°♍51'	07°♋18'	05°♓20'	15°♒01'	22°♐10'
Apr 17 2004	27°♈31'	27°♈14'	11°♊52'	17°♊11'	09°♍24'	07°♋45'	05°♓38'	15°♒08'	22°♐05'
Apr 24 2004	04°♉21'	22°♈42'	17°♊02'	21°♊38'	09°♍05'	08°♋17'	05°♓54'	15°♒14'	21°♐59'
May 1 2004	11°♉09'	21°♈08' D	21°♊19'	26°♊05'	08°♍56'	08°♋52'	06°♓08'	15°♒19'	21°♐52'
May 8 2004	17°♉56'	23°♈23'	24°♊24'	00°♋32'	08°♍55' D	09°♋31'	06°♓20'	15°♒22'	21°♐44'
May 15 2004	24°♉42'	28°♈54'	25°♊59'	04°♋58'	09°♍04'	10°♋13'	06°♓30'	15°♒23'	21°♐35'
May 22 2004	01°♊26'	06°♉58'	25°♊46' ℞	09°♋23'	09°♍21'	10°♋58'	06°♓38'	15°♒23' ℞	21°♐25'
May 29 2004	08°♊09'	17°♉11'	23°♊36'	13°♋49'	09°♍46'	11°♋45'	06°♓43'	15°♒21'	21°♐15'
Jun 5 2004	14°♊52'	29°♉23'	19°♊51'	18°♋14'	10°♍19'	12°♋35'	06°♓47'	15°♒18'	21°♐04'
Jun 12 2004	21°♊33'	13°♊25'	15°♊30'	22°♋39'	11°♍00'	13°♋26'	06°♓47' ℞	15°♒13'	20°♐53'
Jun 19 2004	28°♊15'	28°♊38'	11°♊53'	27°♋03'	11°♍47'	14°♋19'	06°♓46'	15°♒07'	20°♐41'
Jun 26 2004	04°♋55'	13°♋40'	09°♊54'	01°♌28'	12°♍41'	15°♋12'	06°♓41'	14°♒59'	20°♐31'
Jul 3 2004	11°♋36'	27°♋25'	09°♊49' D	05°♌52'	13°♍40'	16°♋07'	06°♓35'	14°♒51'	20°♐20'
Jul 10 2004	18°♋16'	09°♌31'	11°♊30'	10°♌17'	14°♍45'	17°♋01'	06°♓27'	14°♒41'	20°♐10'
Jul 17 2004	24°♋57'	19°♌57'	14°♊39'	14°♌42'	15°♍54'	17°♋56'	06°♓17'	14°♒31'	20°♐01'
Jul 24 2004	01°♌38'	28°♌33'	18°♊54'	19°♌07'	17°♍07'	18°♋50'	06°♓05'	14°♒20'	19°♐53'
Jul 31 2004	08°♌19'	04°♍57'	24°♊00'	23°♌32'	18°♍24'	19°♋43'	05°♓51'	14°♒09'	19°♐46'
Aug 7 2004	15°♌01'	08°♍25'	29°♊46'	27°♌57'	19°♍45'	20°♋35'	05°♓36'	13°♒57'	19°♐41'
Aug 14 2004	21°♌44'	07°♍58' ℞	06°♋04'	02°♍23'	21°♍08'	21°♋25'	05°♓20'	13°♒46'	19°♐36'
Aug 21 2004	28°♌28'	03°♍23'	12°♋46'	06°♍50'	22°♍33'	22°♋14'	05°♓04'	13°♒35'	19°♐33'
Aug 28 2004	05°♍13'	27°♌35'	19°♋48'	11°♍17'	24°♍00'	23°♋00'	04°♓47'	13°♒24'	19°♐32'
Sep 4 2004	12°♍00'	25°♌56' D	27°♋06'	15°♍45'	25°♍29'	23°♋44'	04°♓31'	13°♒14'	19°♐32' D
Sep 11 2004	18°♍47'	00°♍59'	04°♌37'	20°♍14'	26°♍59'	24°♋25'	04°♓14'	13°♒05'	19°♐34'
Sep 18 2004	25°♍37'	11°♍16'	12°♌20'	24°♍43'	28°♍30'	25°♋02'	03°♓59'	12°♒57'	19°♐37'
Sep 25 2004	02°♎28'	23°♍47'	20°♌13'	29°♍14'	00°♎00'	25°♋36'	03°♓44'	12°♒50'	19°♐42'
Oct 2 2004	09°♎20'	06°♎32'	28°♌14'	03°♎45'	01°♎31'	26°♋05'	03°♓31'	12°♒44'	19°♐49'
Oct 9 2004	16°♎14'	18°♎46'	06°♍23'	08°♎18'	03°♎01'	26°♋30'	03°♓19'	12°♒40'	19°♐57'
Oct 16 2004	23°♎10'	00°♏24'	14°♍39'	12°♎52'	04°♎30'	26°♋50'	03°♓09'	12°♒37'	20°♐06'
Oct 23 2004	00°♏07'	11°♏29'	23°♍00'	17°♎27'	05°♎58'	27°♋06'	03°♓01'	12°♒36'	20°♐17'

EST +05:00 Tropical Geo Long	The Sun ☉	Mercury ☿	Venus ♀	Mars ♂	Jupiter ♃	Saturn ♄	Uranus ♅	Neptune ♆	Pluto ♇
Oct 30 2004	07°♏06'	22°♏06'	01°♎25'	22°♎03'	07°♎23'	27°♋15'	02°♓56'	12°♒36' D	20°♐29'
Nov 6 2004	14°♏07'	02°♐16'	09°♎55'	26°♎40'	08°♎47'	27°♋20'	02°♓53'	12°♒39'	20°♐42'
Nov 13 2004	21°♏09'	11°♐50'	18°♎29'	01°♏19'	10°♎07'	27°♋19' ℞	02°♓52' D	12°♒43'	20°♐55'
Nov 20 2004	28°♏13'	20°♐14'	27°♎05'	05°♏59'	11°♎24'	27°♋12'	02°♓54'	12°♒48'	21°♐10'
Nov 27 2004	05°♐17'	25°♐54'	05°♏44'	10°♏41'	12°♎36'	27°♋00'	02°♓58'	12°♒55'	21°♐25'
Dec 4 2004	12°♐23'	25°♐31' ℞	14°♏25'	15°♏23'	13°♎44'	26°♋43'	03°♓05'	13°♒04'	21°♐40'
Dec 11 2004	19°♐29'	17°♐26'	23°♏08'	20°♏08'	14°♎47'	26°♋21'	03°♓14'	13°♒14'	21°♐56'
Dec 18 2004	26°♐37'	10°♐48'	01°♐51'	24°♏53'	15°♎44'	25°♋56'	03°♓25'	13°♒25'	22°♐12'
Dec 25 2004	03°♑44'	12°♐11' D	10°♐36'	29°♏41'	16°♎35'	25°♋26'	03°♓39'	13°♒37'	22°♐28'

Table 14.2 • Position of the Moon 2000–2005

EST +05:00 Tropical Geo Long	The Moon ☽
Jan 1 2000	09°♏48'
Jan 3 2000	03°♐41'
Jan 5 2000	27°♐20'
Jan 7 2000	21°♑05'
Jan 9 2000	15°♒10'
Jan 11 2000	09°♓53'
Jan 13 2000	05°♈33'
Jan 15 2000	02°♉31'
Jan 17 2000	00°♊58'
Jan 19 2000	00°♋37'
Jan 21 2000	00°♌38'
Jan 23 2000	29°♌55'
Jan 25 2000	27°♍41'
Jan 27 2000	23°♎43'
Jan 29 2000	18°♏22'
Jan 31 2000	12°♐12'
Feb 2 2000	05°♑50'
Feb 4 2000	29°♑44'
Feb 6 2000	24°♒15'
Feb 8 2000	19°♓34'
Feb 10 2000	15°♈47'
Feb 12 2000	12°♉55'
Feb 14 2000	10°♊59'
Feb 16 2000	09°♋50'
Feb 18 2000	09°♌00'
Feb 20 2000	07°♍46'
Feb 22 2000	05°♎26'
Feb 24 2000	01°♏36'
Feb 26 2000	26°♏23'
Feb 28 2000	20°♐16'
Mar 1 2000	13°♑55'
Mar 3 2000	07°♒58'
Mar 5 2000	02°♓54'
Mar 7 2000	28°♓57'
Mar 9 2000	25°♈59'
Mar 11 2000	23°♉43'
Mar 13 2000	21°♊50'
Mar 15 2000	20°♋08'
Mar 17 2000	18°♌24'
Mar 19 2000	16°♍20'
Mar 21 2000	13°♎28'
Mar 23 2000	09°♏26'
Mar 25 2000	04°♐12'
Mar 27 2000	28°♐06'
Mar 29 2000	21°♑45'
Mar 31 2000	15°♒53'
Apr 2 2000	11°♓05'
Apr 4 2000	07°♈42'
Apr 6 2000	05°♉36'
Apr 8 2000	04°♊12'
Apr 10 2000	02°♋48'
Apr 12 2000	01°♌00'
Apr 14 2000	28°♌41'
Apr 16 2000	25°♍46'
Apr 18 2000	22°♎09'
Apr 20 2000	17°♏38'
Apr 22 2000	12°♐11'
Apr 24 2000	06°♑01'
Apr 26 2000	29°♑39'
Apr 28 2000	23°♒46'
Apr 30 2000	19°♓02'
May 2 2000	15°♈58'
May 4 2000	14°♉29'

EST +05:00 Tropical Geo Long	The Moon ☽
May 6 2000	13°♊54'
May 8 2000	13°♋14'
May 10 2000	11°♌45'
May 12 2000	09°♍13'
May 14 2000	05°♎45'
May 16 2000	01°♏26'
May 18 2000	26°♏21'
May 20 2000	20°♐34'
May 22 2000	14°♑16'
May 24 2000	07°♒53'
May 26 2000	01°♓59'
May 28 2000	27°♓12'
May 30 2000	24°♈08'
Jun 1 2000	22°♉51'
Jun 3 2000	22°♊46'
Jun 5 2000	22°♋46'
Jun 7 2000	21°♌49'
Jun 9 2000	19°♍27'
Jun 11 2000	15°♎45'
Jun 13 2000	10°♏57'
Jun 15 2000	05°♐23'
Jun 17 2000	29°♐17'
Jun 19 2000	22°♑54'
Jun 21 2000	16°♒34'
Jun 23 2000	10°♓44'
Jun 25 2000	05°♈56'
Jun 27 2000	02°♉41'
Jun 29 2000	01°♊13'
Jul 1 2000	01°♋10'
Jul 3 2000	01°♌29'
Jul 5 2000	01°♍01'
Jul 7 2000	29°♍00'
Jul 9 2000	25°♎19'
Jul 11 2000	20°♏19'
Jul 13 2000	14°♐27'
Jul 15 2000	08°♑08'
Jul 17 2000	01°♒45'
Jul 19 2000	25°♒36'
Jul 21 2000	20°♓01'
Jul 23 2000	15°♈21'
Jul 25 2000	11°♉59'
Jul 27 2000	10°♊08'
Jul 29 2000	09°♋39'
Jul 31 2000	09°♌49'
Aug 2 2000	09°♍30'
Aug 4 2000	07°♎45'
Aug 6 2000	04°♏15'
Aug 8 2000	29°♏14'
Aug 10 2000	23°♐14'
Aug 12 2000	16°♑50'
Aug 14 2000	10°♒33'
Aug 16 2000	04°♓44'
Aug 18 2000	29°♓37'
Aug 20 2000	25°♈20'
Aug 22 2000	22°♉03'
Aug 24 2000	19°♊53'
Aug 26 2000	18°♋47'
Aug 28 2000	18°♌20'
Aug 30 2000	17°♍43'
Sep 1 2000	15°♎58'
Sep 3 2000	12°♏34'
Sep 5 2000	07°♐36'
Sep 7 2000	01°♑35'

EST +05:00 Tropical Geo Long	The Moon ☽
Sep 9 2000	25°♑12'
Sep 11 2000	19°♒04'
Sep 13 2000	13°♓38'
Sep 15 2000	09°♈08'
Sep 17 2000	05°♉31'
Sep 19 2000	02°♊39'
Sep 21 2000	00°♋26'
Sep 23 2000	28°♋48'
Sep 25 2000	27°♌35'
Sep 27 2000	26°♍15'
Sep 29 2000	24°♎05'
Oct 1 2000	20°♏33'
Oct 3 2000	15°♐34'
Oct 5 2000	09°♑33'
Oct 7 2000	03°♒10'
Oct 9 2000	27°♒09'
Oct 11 2000	22°♓03'
Oct 13 2000	18°♈09'
Oct 15 2000	15°♉21'
Oct 17 2000	13°♊14'
Oct 19 2000	11°♋23'
Oct 21 2000	09°♌34'
Oct 23 2000	07°♍40'
Oct 25 2000	05°♎27'
Oct 27 2000	02°♏33'
Oct 29 2000	28°♏35'
Oct 31 2000	23°♐26'
Nov 2 2000	17°♑22'
Nov 4 2000	10°♒59'
Nov 6 2000	04°♓57'
Nov 8 2000	29°♓59'
Nov 10 2000	26°♈28'
Nov 12 2000	24°♉22'
Nov 14 2000	23°♊09'
Nov 16 2000	22°♋03'
Nov 18 2000	20°♌30'
Nov 20 2000	18°♍18'
Nov 22 2000	15°♎22'
Nov 24 2000	11°♏38'
Nov 26 2000	07°♐01'
Nov 28 2000	01°♑32'
Nov 30 2000	25°♑21'
Dec 2 2000	18°♒56'
Dec 4 2000	12°♓51'
Dec 6 2000	07°♈47'
Dec 8 2000	04°♉17'
Dec 10 2000	02°♊30'
Dec 12 2000	01°♋59'
Dec 14 2000	01°♌45'
Dec 16 2000	00°♍54'
Dec 18 2000	28°♍54'
Dec 20 2000	25°♎33'
Dec 22 2000	21°♏10'
Dec 24 2000	15°♐55'
Dec 26 2000	10°♑02'
Dec 28 2000	03°♒43'
Dec 30 2000	27°♒18'
Jan 1 2001	21°♓14'
Jan 3 2001	16°♈01'
Jan 5 2001	12°♉16'
Jan 7 2001	10°♊17'
Jan 9 2001	09°♋55'
Jan 11 2001	10°♌18'

EST +05:00 Tropical Geo Long	The Moon ☽
Jan 13 2001	10°♍11'
Jan 15 2001	08°♎39'
Jan 17 2001	05°♏25'
Jan 19 2001	00°♐43'
Jan 21 2001	25°♐02'
Jan 23 2001	18°♑49'
Jan 25 2001	12°♒25'
Jan 27 2001	06°♓07'
Jan 29 2001	00°♈13'
Jan 31 2001	25°♈02'
Feb 2 2001	21°♉02'
Feb 4 2001	18°♊36'
Feb 6 2001	17°♋51'
Feb 8 2001	18°♌11'
Feb 10 2001	18°♍28'
Feb 12 2001	17°♎26'
Feb 14 2001	14°♏30'
Feb 16 2001	09°♐49'
Feb 18 2001	03°♑59'
Feb 20 2001	27°♑36'
Feb 22 2001	21°♒12'
Feb 24 2001	15°♓08'
Feb 26 2001	09°♈35'
Feb 28 2001	04°♉43'
Mar 2 2001	00°♊46'
Mar 4 2001	28°♊01'
Mar 6 2001	26°♋38'
Mar 8 2001	26°♌24'
Mar 10 2001	26°♍25'
Mar 12 2001	25°♎29'
Mar 14 2001	22°♏47'
Mar 16 2001	18°♐16'
Mar 18 2001	12°♑28'
Mar 20 2001	06°♒05'
Mar 22 2001	29°♒46'
Mar 24 2001	23°♓58'
Mar 26 2001	18°♈55'
Mar 28 2001	14°♉38'
Mar 30 2001	11°♊07'
Apr 1 2001	08°♋24'
Apr 3 2001	06°♌36'
Apr 5 2001	05°♍37'
Apr 7 2001	04°♎53'
Apr 9 2001	03°♏29'
Apr 11 2001	00°♐40'
Apr 13 2001	26°♐13'
Apr 15 2001	20°♑30'
Apr 17 2001	14°♒11'
Apr 19 2001	07°♓59'
Apr 21 2001	02°♈26'
Apr 23 2001	27°♈52'
Apr 25 2001	24°♉17'
Apr 27 2001	21°♊29'
Apr 29 2001	19°♋14'
May 1 2001	17°♌25'
May 3 2001	15°♍52'
May 5 2001	14°♎15'
May 7 2001	12°♏02'
May 9 2001	08°♐42'
May 11 2001	04°♑03'
May 13 2001	28°♑20'
May 15 2001	22°♒05'
May 17 2001	15°♓56'

EST +05:00 Tropical Geo Long	The Moon ☽
May 19 2001	10°♈32'
May 21 2001	06°♉18'
May 23 2001	03°♊19'
May 25 2001	01°♋21'
May 27 2001	29°♋53'
May 29 2001	28°♌26'
May 31 2001	26°♍41'
Jun 2 2001	24°♎22'
Jun 4 2001	21°♏15'
Jun 6 2001	17°♐12'
Jun 8 2001	12°♑10'
Jun 10 2001	06°♒19'
Jun 12 2001	00°♓03'
Jun 14 2001	23°♓55'
Jun 16 2001	18°♈31'
Jun 18 2001	14°♉23'
Jun 20 2001	11°♊46'
Jun 22 2001	10°♋29'
Jun 24 2001	09°♌52'
Jun 26 2001	09°♍05'
Jun 28 2001	07°♎29'
Jun 30 2001	04°♏46'
Jul 2 2001	00°♐57'
Jul 4 2001	26°♐12'
Jul 6 2001	20°♑41'
Jul 8 2001	14°♒38'
Jul 10 2001	08°♓21'
Jul 12 2001	02°♈12'
Jul 14 2001	26°♈44'
Jul 16 2001	22°♉30'
Jul 18 2001	19°♊55'
Jul 20 2001	18°♋58'
Jul 22 2001	19°♌01'
Jul 24 2001	18°♍57'
Jul 26 2001	17°♎44'
Jul 28 2001	14°♏57'
Jul 30 2001	10°♐43'
Aug 1 2001	05°♑28'
Aug 3 2001	29°♑33'
Aug 5 2001	23°♒20'
Aug 7 2001	17°♓03'
Aug 9 2001	10°♈58'
Aug 11 2001	05°♉30'
Aug 13 2001	01°♊06'
Aug 15 2001	28°♊17'
Aug 17 2001	27°♋15'
Aug 19 2001	27°♌32'
Aug 21 2001	27°♍56'
Aug 23 2001	27°♎09'
Aug 25 2001	24°♏30'
Aug 27 2001	20°♐11'
Aug 29 2001	14°♑39'
Aug 31 2001	08°♒31'
Sep 2 2001	02°♓12'
Sep 4 2001	26°♓01'
Sep 6 2001	20°♈09'
Sep 8 2001	14°♉51'
Sep 10 2001	10°♊26'
Sep 12 2001	07°♋21'
Sep 14 2001	05°♌55'
Sep 16 2001	05°♍54'
Sep 18 2001	06°♎18'
Sep 20 2001	05°♏43'
Sep 22 2001	03°♐19'
Sep 24 2001	29°♐03'
Sep 26 2001	23°♑29'
Sep 28 2001	17°♒16'
Sep 30 2001	10°♓58'
Oct 2 2001	04°♈58'
Oct 4 2001	29°♈28'
Oct 6 2001	24°♉34'
Oct 8 2001	20°♊26'
Oct 10 2001	17°♋19'
Oct 12 2001	15°♌28'
Oct 14 2001	14°♍49'
Oct 16 2001	14°♎38'
Oct 18 2001	13°♏48'
Oct 20 2001	11°♐25'
Oct 22 2001	07°♑16'
Oct 24 2001	01°♒47'
Oct 26 2001	25°♒36'
Oct 28 2001	19°♓21'
Oct 30 2001	13°♈34'
Nov 1 2001	08°♉30'
Nov 3 2001	04°♊14'
Nov 5 2001	00°♋42'
Nov 7 2001	27°♋57'
Nov 9 2001	25°♌58'
Nov 11 2001	24°♍39'
Nov 13 2001	23°♎34'
Nov 15 2001	22°♏00'
Nov 17 2001	19°♐15'
Nov 19 2001	15°♑04'
Nov 21 2001	09°♒39'
Nov 23 2001	03°♓31'
Nov 25 2001	27°♓19'
Nov 27 2001	21°♈39'
Nov 29 2001	16°♉55'
Dec 1 2001	13°♊17'
Dec 3 2001	10°♋38'
Dec 5 2001	08°♌39'
Dec 7 2001	06°♍59'
Dec 9 2001	05°♎20'
Dec 11 2001	03°♏23'
Dec 13 2001	00°♐51'
Dec 15 2001	27°♐24'
Dec 17 2001	22°♑54'
Dec 19 2001	17°♒26'
Dec 21 2001	11°♓19'
Dec 23 2001	05°♈06'
Dec 25 2001	29°♈22'
Dec 27 2001	24°♉44'
Dec 29 2001	21°♊31'
Dec 31 2001	19°♋41'
Jan 2 2002	18°♌42'
Jan 4 2002	17°♍48'
Jan 6 2002	16°♎17'
Jan 8 2002	13°♏50'
Jan 10 2002	10°♐27'
Jan 12 2002	06°♑18'
Jan 14 2002	01°♒11'
Jan 16 2002	25°♒30'
Jan 18 2002	19°♓20'
Jan 20 2002	13°♈04'
Jan 22 2002	07°♉14'
Jan 24 2002	02°♊27'
Jan 26 2002	29°♊15'
Jan 28 2002	27°♋51'
Jan 30 2002	27°♌42'
Feb 1 2002	27°♍41'
Feb 3 2002	26°♎43'
Feb 5 2002	24°♏15'
Feb 7 2002	20°♐24'
Feb 9 2002	15°♑32'
Feb 11 2002	10°♒00'
Feb 13 2002	04°♓02'
Feb 15 2002	27°♓49'
Feb 17 2002	21°♈33'
Feb 19 2002	15°♉39'
Feb 21 2002	10°♊40'
Feb 23 2002	07°♋13'
Feb 25 2002	05°♌44'
Feb 27 2002	05°♍52'
Mar 1 2002	06°♎29'
Mar 3 2002	06°♏08'
Mar 5 2002	04°♐00'
Mar 7 2002	00°♑06'
Mar 9 2002	24°♑57'
Mar 11 2002	19°♒05'
Mar 13 2002	12°♓54'
Mar 15 2002	06°♈39'
Mar 17 2002	00°♉29'
Mar 19 2002	24°♉42'
Mar 21 2002	19°♊42'
Mar 23 2002	16°♋03'
Mar 25 2002	14°♌04'
Mar 27 2002	14°♍01'
Mar 29 2002	14°♎38'
Mar 31 2002	14°♏35'
Apr 2 2002	12°♐48'
Apr 4 2002	09°♑08'
Apr 6 2002	04°♒01'
Apr 8 2002	28°♒02'
Apr 10 2002	21°♓45'
Apr 12 2002	15°♈32'
Apr 14 2002	09°♉31'
Apr 16 2002	04°♊10'
Apr 18 2002	29°♊27'
Apr 20 2002	25°♋50'
Apr 22 2002	23°♌40'
Apr 24 2002	22°♍55'
Apr 26 2002	22°♎58'
Apr 28 2002	22°♏38'
Apr 30 2002	20°♐56'
May 2 2002	17°♑28'
May 4 2002	12°♒30'
May 6 2002	06°♓35'
May 8 2002	00°♈19'
May 10 2002	24°♈12'
May 12 2002	18°♉34'
May 14 2002	13°♊38'
May 16 2002	09°♋30'
May 18 2002	06°♌18'
May 20 2002	04°♍07'
May 22 2002	02°♎50'
May 24 2002	02°♏03'
May 26 2002	00°♐59'
May 28 2002	28°♐55'
May 30 2002	25°♑25'
Jun 1 2002	20°♒32'
Jun 3 2002	14°♓42'
Jun 5 2002	08°♈29'
Jun 7 2002	02°♉28'
Jun 9 2002	27°♉07'
Jun 11 2002	22°♊44'
Jun 13 2002	19°♋23'
Jun 15 2002	16°♌55'
Jun 17 2002	15°♍05'
Jun 19 2002	13°♎33'
Jun 21 2002	12°♏00'
Jun 23 2002	10°♐02'
Jun 25 2002	07°♑16'
Jun 27 2002	03°♒25'
Jun 29 2002	28°♒28'
Jul 1 2002	22°♓38'
Jul 3 2002	16°♈26'
Jul 5 2002	10°♉26'
Jul 7 2002	05°♊18'
Jul 9 2002	01°♋20'
Jul 11 2002	28°♋45'
Jul 13 2002	27°♌12'
Jul 15 2002	26°♍01'
Jul 17 2002	24°♎35'
Jul 19 2002	22°♏32'
Jul 21 2002	19°♐45'
Jul 23 2002	16°♑12'
Jul 25 2002	11°♒49'
Jul 27 2002	06°♓35'
Jul 29 2002	00°♈40'
Jul 31 2002	24°♈25'
Aug 2 2002	18°♉22'
Aug 4 2002	13°♊12'
Aug 6 2002	09°♋29'
Aug 8 2002	07°♌28'
Aug 10 2002	06°♍45'
Aug 12 2002	06°♎22'
Aug 14 2002	05°♏21'
Aug 16 2002	03°♐10'
Aug 18 2002	29°♐51'
Aug 20 2002	25°♑38'
Aug 22 2002	20°♒41'
Aug 24 2002	15°♓06'
Aug 26 2002	09°♈01'
Aug 28 2002	02°♉42'
Aug 30 2002	26°♉35'
Sep 1 2002	21°♊19'
Sep 3 2002	17°♋34'
Sep 5 2002	15°♌43'
Sep 7 2002	15°♍29'
Sep 9 2002	15°♎48'
Sep 11 2002	15°♏21'
Sep 13 2002	13°♐23'
Sep 15 2002	09°♑54'
Sep 17 2002	05°♒15'
Sep 19 2002	29°♒51'
Sep 21 2002	23°♓56'
Sep 23 2002	17°♈43'
Sep 25 2002	11°♉23'
Sep 27 2002	05°♊18'
Sep 29 2002	29°♊11'
Oct 1 2002	26°♋04'
Oct 3 2002	24°♌01'

EST +05:00 Tropical Geo Long	The Moon ☽
Oct 5 2002	23°♍45'
Oct 7 2002	24°♎19'
Oct 9 2002	24°♏19'
Oct 11 2002	22°♐45'
Oct 13 2002	19°♑25'
Oct 15 2002	14°♒39'
Oct 17 2002	08°♓59'
Oct 19 2002	02°♈51'
Oct 21 2002	26°♈34'
Oct 23 2002	20°♉22'
Oct 25 2002	14°♊30'
Oct 27 2002	09°♋20'
Oct 29 2002	05°♌21'
Oct 31 2002	02°♍58'
Nov 2 2002	02°♎12'
Nov 4 2002	02°♏25'
Nov 6 2002	02°♐27'
Nov 8 2002	01°♑10'
Nov 10 2002	28°♑08'
Nov 12 2002	23°♒30'
Nov 14 2002	17°♓46'
Nov 16 2002	11°♈32'
Nov 18 2002	05°♉15'
Nov 20 2002	29°♉17'
Nov 22 2002	23°♊51'
Nov 24 2002	19°♋11'
Nov 26 2002	15°♌28'
Nov 28 2002	12°♍54'
Nov 30 2002	11°♎30'
Dec 2 2002	10°♏56'
Dec 4 2002	10°♐24'
Dec 6 2002	09°♑00'
Dec 8 2002	06°♒07'
Dec 10 2002	01°♓41'
Dec 12 2002	26°♓02'
Dec 14 2002	19°♈47'
Dec 16 2002	13°♉32'
Dec 18 2002	07°♊48'
Dec 20 2002	02°♋55'
Dec 22 2002	29°♋00'
Dec 24 2002	25°♌57'
Dec 26 2002	23°♍38'
Dec 28 2002	21°♎52'
Dec 30 2002	20°♏27'
Jan 1 2003	18°♐59'
Jan 3 2003	16°♑59'
Jan 5 2003	13°♒53'
Jan 7 2003	09°♓28'
Jan 9 2003	03°♈53'
Jan 11 2003	27°♈38'
Jan 13 2003	21°♉23'
Jan 15 2003	15°♊49'
Jan 17 2003	11°♋23'
Jan 19 2003	08°♌15'
Jan 21 2003	06°♍09'
Jan 23 2003	04°♎31'
Jan 25 2003	02°♏51'
Jan 27 2003	00°♐55'
Jan 29 2003	28°♐34'
Jan 31 2003	25°♑41'
Feb 2 2003	22°♒01'
Feb 4 2003	17°♓20'
Feb 6 2003	11°♈41'

EST +05:00 Tropical Geo Long	The Moon ☽
Feb 8 2003	05°♉25'
Feb 10 2003	29°♉07'
Feb 12 2003	23°♊32'
Feb 14 2003	19°♋18'
Feb 16 2003	16°♌43'
Feb 18 2003	15°♍29'
Feb 20 2003	14°♎46'
Feb 22 2003	13°♏40'
Feb 24 2003	11°♐42'
Feb 26 2003	08°♑51'
Feb 28 2003	05°♒12'
Mar 2 2003	00°♓49'
Mar 4 2003	25°♓41'
Mar 6 2003	19°♈49'
Mar 8 2003	13°♉28'
Mar 10 2003	07°♊07'
Mar 12 2003	01°♋27'
Mar 14 2003	27°♋09'
Mar 16 2003	24°♌42'
Mar 18 2003	23°♍56'
Mar 20 2003	23°♎59'
Mar 22 2003	23°♏38'
Mar 24 2003	22°♐05'
Mar 26 2003	19°♑09'
Mar 28 2003	15°♒05'
Mar 30 2003	10°♓07'
Apr 1 2003	04°♈29'
Apr 3 2003	28°♈21'
Apr 5 2003	21°♉56'
Apr 7 2003	15°♊37'
Apr 9 2003	09°♋56'
Apr 11 2003	05°♌31'
Apr 13 2003	02°♍52'
Apr 15 2003	02°♎03'
Apr 17 2003	02°♏22'
Apr 19 2003	02°♐34'
Apr 21 2003	01°♑34'
Apr 23 2003	28°♑55'
Apr 25 2003	24°♒45'
Apr 27 2003	19°♓28'
Apr 29 2003	13°♈29'
May 1 2003	07°♉09'
May 3 2003	00°♊46'
May 5 2003	24°♊37'
May 7 2003	19°♋05'
May 9 2003	14°♌40'
May 11 2003	11°♍46'
May 13 2003	10°♎33'
May 15 2003	10°♏35'
May 17 2003	10°♐51'
May 19 2003	10°♑11'
May 21 2003	07°♒53'
May 23 2003	03°♓51'
May 25 2003	28°♓30'
May 27 2003	22°♈21'
May 29 2003	15°♉56'
May 31 2003	09°♊40'
Jun 2 2003	03°♋50'
Jun 4 2003	28°♋43'
Jun 6 2003	24°♌33'
Jun 8 2003	21°♍35'
Jun 10 2003	19°♎54'
Jun 12 2003	19°♏18'

EST +05:00 Tropical Geo Long	The Moon ☽
Jun 14 2003	19°♐08'
Jun 16 2003	18°♑23'
Jun 18 2003	16°♒13'
Jun 20 2003	12°♓21'
Jun 22 2003	07°♈02'
Jun 24 2003	00°♉51'
Jun 26 2003	24°♉27'
Jun 28 2003	18°♊22'
Jun 30 2003	12°♋59'
Jul 2 2003	08°♌29'
Jul 4 2003	04°♍52'
Jul 6 2003	02°♎06'
Jul 8 2003	00°♏10'
Jul 10 2003	28°♏54'
Jul 12 2003	27°♐58'
Jul 14 2003	26°♑41'
Jul 16 2003	24°♒18'
Jul 18 2003	20°♓25'
Jul 20 2003	15°♈08'
Jul 22 2003	08°♉58'
Jul 24 2003	02°♊37'
Jul 26 2003	26°♊44'
Jul 28 2003	21°♋47'
Jul 30 2003	17°♌58'
Aug 1 2003	15°♍07'
Aug 3 2003	12°♎55'
Aug 5 2003	11°♏02'
Aug 7 2003	09°♐20'
Aug 9 2003	07°♑37'
Aug 11 2003	05°♒32'
Aug 13 2003	02°♓35'
Aug 15 2003	28°♓25'
Aug 17 2003	23°♈03'
Aug 19 2003	16°♉52'
Aug 21 2003	10°♊32'
Aug 23 2003	04°♋44'
Aug 25 2003	00°♌06'
Aug 27 2003	26°♌53'
Aug 29 2003	24°♍51'
Aug 31 2003	23°♎26'
Sep 2 2003	22°♏00'
Sep 4 2003	20°♐12'
Sep 6 2003	17°♑55'
Sep 8 2003	15°♒01'
Sep 10 2003	11°♓20'
Sep 12 2003	06°♈41'
Sep 14 2003	01°♉05'
Sep 16 2003	24°♉49'
Sep 18 2003	18°♊27'
Sep 20 2003	12°♋39'
Sep 22 2003	08°♌05'
Sep 24 2003	05°♍09'
Sep 26 2003	03°♎45'
Sep 28 2003	03°♏09'
Sep 30 2003	02°♐27'
Oct 2 2003	00°♑57'
Oct 4 2003	28°♑27'
Oct 6 2003	24°♒57'
Oct 8 2003	20°♓33'
Oct 10 2003	15°♈20'
Oct 12 2003	09°♉23'
Oct 14 2003	03°♊04'
Oct 16 2003	26°♊41'

EST +05:00 Tropical Geo Long	The Moon ☽
Oct 18 2003	20°♋50'
Oct 20 2003	16°♌09'
Oct 22 2003	13°♍09'
Oct 24 2003	11°♎54'
Oct 26 2003	11°♏55'
Oct 28 2003	11°♐53'
Oct 30 2003	11°♑00'
Nov 1 2003	08°♒39'
Nov 3 2003	04°♓53'
Nov 5 2003	29°♓58'
Nov 7 2003	24°♈16'
Nov 9 2003	18°♉04'
Nov 11 2003	11°♊40'
Nov 13 2003	05°♋22'
Nov 15 2003	29°♋35'
Nov 17 2003	24°♌47'
Nov 19 2003	21°♍29'
Nov 21 2003	19°♎55'
Nov 23 2003	19°♏49'
Nov 25 2003	20°♐15'
Nov 27 2003	19°♑57'
Nov 29 2003	18°♒03'
Dec 1 2003	14°♓21'
Dec 3 2003	09°♈13'
Dec 5 2003	03°♉13'
Dec 7 2003	26°♉50'
Dec 9 2003	20°♊29'
Dec 11 2003	14°♋25'
Dec 13 2003	08°♌55'
Dec 15 2003	04°♍13'
Dec 17 2003	00°♎41'
Dec 19 2003	28°♎36'
Dec 21 2003	27°♏58'
Dec 23 2003	28°♐09'
Dec 25 2003	28°♑02'
Dec 27 2003	26°♒29'
Dec 29 2003	23°♓02'
Dec 31 2003	17°♈57'
Jan 2 2004	11°♉51'
Jan 4 2004	05°♊25'
Jan 6 2004	29°♊10'
Jan 8 2004	23°♋29'
Jan 10 2004	18°♌29'
Jan 12 2004	14°♍15'
Jan 14 2004	10°♎50'
Jan 16 2004	08°♏25'
Jan 18 2004	07°♐05'
Jan 20 2004	06°♑32'
Jan 22 2004	05°♒58'
Jan 24 2004	04°♓20'
Jan 26 2004	01°♈01'
Jan 28 2004	26°♈04'
Jan 30 2004	20°♉01'
Feb 1 2004	13°♊36'
Feb 3 2004	07°♋30'
Feb 5 2004	02°♌10'
Feb 7 2004	27°♌48'
Feb 9 2004	24°♍16'
Feb 11 2004	21°♎25'
Feb 13 2004	19°♏07'
Feb 15 2004	17°♐22'
Feb 17 2004	15°♑59'
Feb 19 2004	14°♒33'

EST +05:00 Tropical Geo Long	The Moon ☽
Feb 21 2004	12°♓20'
Feb 23 2004	08°♈47'
Feb 25 2004	03°♉49'
Feb 27 2004	27°♉50'
Feb 29 2004	21°♊29'
Mar 2 2004	15°♋27'
Mar 4 2004	10°♌21'
Mar 6 2004	06°♍29'
Mar 8 2004	03°♎44'
Mar 10 2004	01°♏44'
Mar 12 2004	00°♐01'
Mar 14 2004	28°♐19'
Mar 16 2004	26°♑25'
Mar 18 2004	24°♒04'
Mar 20 2004	20°♓59'
Mar 22 2004	16°♈52'
Mar 24 2004	11°♉40'
Mar 26 2004	05°♊39'
Mar 28 2004	29°♊19'
Mar 30 2004	23°♋18'
Apr 1 2004	18°♌14'
Apr 3 2004	14°♍35'
Apr 5 2004	12°♎24'
Apr 7 2004	11°♏15'
Apr 9 2004	10°♐24'
Apr 11 2004	09°♑11'
Apr 13 2004	07°♒10'
Apr 15 2004	04°♓13'
Apr 17 2004	00°♈19'
Apr 19 2004	25°♈31'
Apr 21 2004	19°♉56'
Apr 23 2004	13°♊47'
Apr 25 2004	07°♋26'
Apr 27 2004	01°♌24'
Apr 29 2004	26°♌16'
May 1 2004	22°♍33'
May 3 2004	20°♎32'
May 5 2004	19°♏56'
May 7 2004	19°♐54'
May 9 2004	19°♑22'

EST +05:00 Tropical Geo Long	The Moon ☽
May 11 2004	17°♒37'
May 13 2004	14°♓25'
May 15 2004	09°♈57'
May 17 2004	04°♉35'
May 19 2004	28°♉37'
May 21 2004	22°♊19'
May 23 2004	16°♋00'
May 25 2004	10°♌00'
May 27 2004	04°♍48'
May 29 2004	00°♎54'
May 31 2004	28°♎43'
Jun 2 2004	28°♏12'
Jun 4 2004	28°♐36'
Jun 6 2004	28°♑40'
Jun 8 2004	27°♒19'
Jun 10 2004	24°♓10'
Jun 12 2004	19°♈29'
Jun 14 2004	13°♉45'
Jun 16 2004	07°♊31'
Jun 18 2004	01°♋10'
Jun 20 2004	24°♋58'
Jun 22 2004	19°♌08'
Jun 24 2004	14°♍01'
Jun 26 2004	09°♎59'
Jun 28 2004	07°♏29'
Jun 30 2004	06°♐39'
Jul 2 2004	06°♑59'
Jul 4 2004	07°♒15'
Jul 6 2004	06°♓13'
Jul 8 2004	03°♈14'
Jul 10 2004	28°♈32'
Jul 12 2004	22°♉42'
Jul 14 2004	16°♊22'
Jul 16 2004	10°♋03'
Jul 18 2004	04°♌04'
Jul 20 2004	28°♌35'
Jul 22 2004	23°♍46'
Jul 24 2004	19°♎50'
Jul 26 2004	17°♏08'
Jul 28 2004	15°♐50'

EST +05:00 Tropical Geo Long	The Moon ☽
Jul 30 2004	15°♑39'
Aug 1 2004	15°♒36'
Aug 3 2004	14°♓31'
Aug 5 2004	11°♈38'
Aug 7 2004	07°♉01'
Aug 9 2004	01°♊13'
Aug 11 2004	24°♊54'
Aug 13 2004	18°♋41'
Aug 15 2004	12°♌59'
Aug 17 2004	07°♍59'
Aug 19 2004	03°♎43'
Aug 21 2004	00°♏13'
Aug 23 2004	27°♏35'
Aug 25 2004	25°♐55'
Aug 27 2004	25°♑02'
Aug 29 2004	24°♒15'
Aug 31 2004	22°♓40'
Sep 2 2004	19°♈38'
Sep 4 2004	15°♉02'
Sep 6 2004	09°♊18'
Sep 8 2004	03°♋02'
Sep 10 2004	26°♋55'
Sep 12 2004	21°♌28'
Sep 14 2004	16°♍57'
Sep 16 2004	13°♎23'
Sep 18 2004	10°♏37'
Sep 20 2004	08°♐28'
Sep 22 2004	06°♑45'
Sep 24 2004	05°♒15'
Sep 26 2004	03°♓33'
Sep 28 2004	01°♈09'
Sep 30 2004	27°♈38'
Oct 2 2004	22°♉53'
Oct 4 2004	17°♊08'
Oct 6 2004	10°♋55'
Oct 8 2004	04°♌50'
Oct 10 2004	29°♌28'
Oct 12 2004	25°♍16'
Oct 14 2004	22°♎22'
Oct 16 2004	20°♏30'

EST +05:00 Tropical Geo Long	The Moon ☽
Oct 18 2004	19°♐09'
Oct 20 2004	17°♑48'
Oct 22 2004	16°♒01'
Oct 24 2004	13°♓32'
Oct 26 2004	10°♈14'
Oct 28 2004	06°♉02'
Oct 30 2004	00°♊55'
Nov 1 2004	25°♊05'
Nov 3 2004	18°♋51'
Nov 5 2004	12°♌42'
Nov 7 2004	07°♍16'
Nov 9 2004	03°♎06'
Nov 11 2004	00°♏32'
Nov 13 2004	29°♏25'
Nov 15 2004	29°♐02'
Nov 17 2004	28°♑24'
Nov 19 2004	26°♒45'
Nov 21 2004	23°♓51'
Nov 23 2004	19°♈50'
Nov 25 2004	14°♉56'
Nov 27 2004	09°♊24'
Nov 29 2004	03°♋23'
Dec 1 2004	27°♋07'
Dec 3 2004	20°♌56'
Dec 5 2004	15°♍21'
Dec 7 2004	10°♎59'
Dec 9 2004	08°♏20'
Dec 11 2004	07°♐30'
Dec 13 2004	07°♑48'
Dec 15 2004	07°♒58'
Dec 17 2004	06°♓49'
Dec 19 2004	03°♈55'
Dec 21 2004	29°♈32'
Dec 23 2004	24°♉10'
Dec 25 2004	18°♊15'
Dec 27 2004	12°♋04'
Dec 29 2004	05°♌49'
Dec 31 2004	29°♌43'

Appendix I

Calculating Your Ascendant, or Rising Sign

To calculate your ascendant—the sign appearing on the horizon at the moment you were born—follow these steps using Table I.*

1. Find your Sun sign in the left-hand column.
2. Read the line across until you find the range of time in which you were born.
3. Once you find the span of time, the rising sign is listed at the top of the column.

Let's say you were born on January 28 at 1:20 P.M. First, read the horizontal line for Aquarius, your Sun sign, on the left-hand side. Read the line across until you find the column listing the

---

* This table only provides an approximation of your rising sign and may not be 100 percent accurate. If you wish to verify the information in the following tables, use the chart services listed in Appendix V.

time span between 1 and 3 P.M. Gemini, the sign at the top of the column, is therefore your ascendant.

If you were born during daylight saving time,† first subtract one hour before looking up your rising sign. Let's say that you were born on June 3 at 3:05 A.M. in New York City. Since New York always adheres to daylight saving time, you would look to the column for Gemini 2:05 A.M., which yields Aries as your rising sign.

---

† *If you were born between April and October, it is necessary to find out if daylight saving time was in effect at the time and place of your birth.*

Appendix I

Table I. Calculating Your Ascendant, or Rising Sign

RISING SIGN	ARIES	TAURUS	GEMINI	CANCER	LEO	VIRGO	LIBRA
Aries	5–7 A.M.	7–9 A.M.	9–11 A.M.	11 A.M.–1 P.M.	1–3 P.M.	3–5 P.M.	5–7 P.M.
Taurus	3–5 A.M.	5–7 A.M.	7–9 A.M.	9–11 A.M.	11 A.M.–1 P.M.	1–3 P.M.	3–5 P.M.
Gemini	1–3 A.M.	3–5 A.M.	5–7 A.M.	7–9 A.M.	9–11 A.M.	11 A.M.–1 P.M.	1–3 P.M.
Cancer	11 P.M.–1 A.M.	1–3 A.M.	3–5 A.M.	5–7 A.M.	7–9 A.M.	9–11 A.M.	11 A.M.–1 P.M.
Leo	9–11 P.M.	11 P.M.–1 A.M.	1–3 A.M.	3–5 A.M.	5–7 A.M.	7–9 A.M.	9–11 A.M.
Virgo	7–9 P.M.	9–11 P.M.	11 P.M.–1 A.M.	1–3 A.M.	3–5 A.M.	5–7 A.M.	7–9 A.M.
Libra	5–7 P.M.	7–9 P.M.	9–11 P.M.	11 P.M.–1 A.M.	1–3 A.M.	3–5 A.M.	5–7 A.M.
Scorpio	3–5 P.M.	5–7 P.M.	7–9 P.M.	9–11 P.M.	11 P.M.–1 A.M.	1–3 A.M.	3–5 A.M.
Sagittarius	1–3 P.M.	3–5 P.M.	5–7 P.M.	7–9 P.M.	9–11 P.M.	11 P.M.–1 A.M.	1–3 A.M.
Capricorn	11 A.M.–1 P.M.	1–3 P.M.	3–5 P.M.	5–7 P.M.	7–9 P.M.	9–11 P.M.	11 P.M.–1 A.M.
Aquarius	9–11 A.M.	11 A.M.–1 P.M.	1–3 P.M.	3–5 P.M.	5–7 P.M.	7–9 P.M.	9–11 P.M.
Pisces	7–9 A.M.	9–11 A.M.	11 A.M.–1 P.M.	1–3 P.M.	3–5 P.M.	5–7 P.M.	7–9 P.M.

RISING SIGN	SCORPIO	SAGITTARIUS	CAPRICORN	AQUARIUS	PISCES
Aries	7–9 P.M.	9–11 P.M.	11 P.M.–1 A.M.	1–3 A.M.	3–5 A.M.
Taurus	5–7 P.M.	7–9 P.M.	9–11 P.M.	11 P.M.–1 A.M.	1–3 A.M.
Gemini	3–5 P.M.	5–7 P.M.	7–9 P.M.	9–11 P.M.	11 P.M.–1 A.M.
Cancer	1–3 P.M.	3–5 P.M.	5–7 P.M.	7–9 P.M.	9–11 P.M.
Leo	11 A.M.–1 P.M.	1–3 P.M.	3–5 P.M.	5–7 P.M.	7–9 P.M.
Virgo	9–11 A.M.	11 A.M.–1 P.M.	1–3 P.M.	3–5 P.M.	5–7 P.M.
Libra	7–9 A.M.	9–11 A.M.	11 A.M.–1 P.M.	1–3 P.M.	3–5 P.M.
Scorpio	5–7 A.M.	7–9 A.M.	9–11 A.M.	11 A.M.–1 P.M.	1–3 P.M.
Sagittarius	3–5 A.M.	5–7 A.M.	7–9 A.M.	9–11 A.M.	11 A.M.–1 P.M.
Capricorn	1–3 A.M.	3–5 A.M.	5–7 A.M.	7–9 A.M.	9–11 A.M.
Aquarius	11 P.M.–1 A.M.	1–3 A.M.	3–5 A.M.	5–7 A.M.	7–9 A.M.
Pisces	9–11 P.M.	11 P.M.–1 A.M.	1–3 A.M.	3–5 A.M.	5–7 A.M.

Holistic Healing Techniques

⁕

The techniques discussed throughout this book will restore the body's natural balance by preventing the onset of, and providing relief from, those conditions which may be a by-product of an unhealthy and/or stressful lifestyle. Always consult your doctor before starting a new diet or strenuous exercise plan. If you are at risk for or suffer from a serious, chronic, or life-threatening illness, do not forego orthodox, or allopathic, treatment in favor of a completely holistic cure. If you get the green light from your doctor, however, these methods may be used in conjunction with traditional treatment and medication. While orthodox medicine and drug therapy are invaluable for fighting certain infections and other acute illnesses, alternative treatment offers relief from stress, stress-induced problems, and chronic ailments such as arthritis, osteoporosis, asthma, backache, and others mentioned throughout this book.

DIET AND NUTRITION

Nutrition is the relationship between how food nourishes, energizes, and keeps the body healthy. Nutritional counseling is the process of prescribing the proper balance of nutrients to prevent or fight illness since the right amount of vitamins, minerals, and amino acids strengthens the overall immune system, and is beneficial to the blood, general vitality, and very specific areas of the body. In addition to obtaining these nutrients from a balanced diet, vitamin and mineral supplements can supply the Recommended Dietary Allowance (RDA)* needed for good health and to prevent certain nutritional deficiencies.

Some foods are beneficial for disease prevention while others cause or exacerbate existing ailments. For instance, high-cholesterol foods are detrimental to the heart, fatty foods aggravate gallstones, alcohol damages the liver, and sugar is deadly for diabetics. By the same token, fiber heals the colon, and water flushes the kidneys.

Although medical school does not require a curriculum that includes nutrition (believe it or not), many medical practitioners are beginning to realize that proper nutrition plays a significant role in promoting good health and proper functioning of organs. Conversely, a poor diet interferes with the healing process and is, in part, responsible for heart ailments, diabetes, liver ailments, kidney problems, and intestinal difficulties. If you are genetically predisposed to these illnesses, proper diet can, in some cases, prevent their onset.

Since different nutrients are especially beneficial for each zodiacal sign and the organs/ailments it represents, it is useful to

---

* RDAs are guidelines set by the U.S. Food and Drug Administration as to the daily dosage of vitamins and minerals recommended for good health.

explain how each nutrient affects the body and which foods supply them.

VITAMINS

Vitamins are chemicals which the body cannot manufacture yet requires for proper growth, repair, and other vital functions. Vitamins fall into two categories—fat soluble (carried through the blood in fat) and water soluble (carried through the blood by water). Since specific foods supply concentrations of certain vitamins, the inclusion of a wide variety of nutrients will provide the majority of the essential ones. For the most part, raw, fresh fruits and vegetables are the best sources of vitamins and minerals, especially the skins; cooking and boiling destroys vitamins. Table A lists vitamins, their purpose, foods which supply them, and results of deficiency.

TABLE A—VITAMINS

VITAMINS	FAT OR WATER SOLUBLE	BODILY FUNCTION	FOODS PROVIDING VITAMINS	RDA RESULTS OF DEFICIENCY
Vitamin A (Carotene)	Fat soluble	Maintenance of healthy skin, eyes, bones, hair, and teeth. Good eyesight. Growth and repair of body tissues.	Carrots, beets, greens, spinach, broccoli, fish liver oil	1000 RE* for men and 800 RE for women. Night blindness; rough, dry, scaly skin; frequent fatigue; loss of appetite
Vitamin B$_1$ (Thiamine)	Water soluble	Strengthens nervous system; needed for normal appetite; stimulates growth and muscle tone	Whole grains, oatmeal, legumes and other beans, potatoes, lean meats and fish	1.5 mg for men and 1.1 mg for women. Fatigue; loss of appetite; weak nervous system; gastrointestinal disorders
Vitamin B$_2$ (Riboflavin)	Water soluble	Maintains healthy skin and eyes; Aids in formation of antibodies and red blood cells.	Liver, meat, eggs, beans, nuts, and dairy products	1.7 mg for men and 1.3 mg for women. Skin rashes; digestive disorders
Vitamin B$_3$ (Niacin)	Water soluble	Maintains healthy skin and digestive system and strengthens nervous system	Breads, peanuts, potatoes, broadbeans, and chocolate	19 mg for men and 15 mg for women. Weakened nervous system; skin sensitivities

* Retinol equivalent

VITAMINS	FAT OR WATER SOLUBLE	BODILY FUNCTION	FOODS PROVIDING VITAMINS	RDA RESULTS OF DEFICIENCY
Vitamin B_6 (Pyridoxine)	*Water soluble*	*Necessary to control the nervous system; assists protein and fat metabolism; essential for function of red blood cells and formation of antibodies*	*Bananas, peanuts, fish, liver, potatoes, raisins*	*2 mg for males 1.6 mg for females. Weak nervous system; muscular weakness, skin sensitivities*
Vitamin B_{12} (Cyanocobalamin)	*Water soluble*	*Prevents pernicious anemia; necessary for healthy nervous system; synthesizes genetic material (DNA)*	*Milk, meat, eggs, and fish*	*2 mcg for males and females. Weak nervous system; anemia*
Biotin	*Water soluble*	*Aids in utilization of other B vitamins; needed for normal hair production and growth*	*Most vegetables, liver and kidneys, milk, cheddar cheese, canned salmon*	*30–100 mg for males and females. Sensitive skin; skin allergies; depression; lack of appetite; unable to metabolize fats*
Choline	*Water soluble*	*Regulates the metabolism and breakdown of fats; strengthens nerves*	*Egg yolk, liver, brewer's yeast, wheat germ*	*No RDA. High blood pressure; poor liver and gallbladder functioning*

VITAMINS	FAT OR WATER SOLUBLE	BODILY FUNCTION	FOODS PROVIDING VITAMINS	RDA RESULTS OF DEFICIENCY
Folic acid	Water soluble	Necessary for red blood cell formation; helps metabolize fats and amino acids; necessary for growth and division of body cells	Meats, fruits, vegetables	200 mcg for men and women. Gastrointestinal disorders; anemia
Inositol	Water soluble	Helps metabolize fats and cholesterol; necessary for healthy hair	Whole grains, citrus fruits, brewer's yeast, unrefined molasses, liver	No RDA. Skin problems; hair thinning and possible loss; high cholesterol
Pantothenic acid	Water soluble	Needed for normal functioning of the adrenal glands	Liver, kidneys, milk, raw mushrooms, egg yolk, cereals	4–7 mg for males and females. Listlessness; nausea; weakened immune system
Vitamin C (ascorbic acid)	Water soluble	Maintains bones, teeth, and blood vessels; enhances iron absorption and red blood cell formation; heals wounds and strengthens immune system	Oranges, lemons, grapefruit, broccoli, sprouts, peppers, strawberries	60 mg for men and women. Susceptible to colds; bleeding gums; painful joints; slow healing process; nosebleeds

VITAMINS	FAT OR WATER SOLUBLE	BODILY FUNCTION	FOODS PROVIDING VITAMINS	RDA RESULTS OF DEFICIENCY
Vitamin D	*Fat soluble*	*Assists in the absorption and metabolism of calcium and phosphorus for strong bones and teeth*	*Fortified milk, fish liver oils*	*200 IU* for men and women. Weak bones, teeth, and skin*
Vitamin E	*Fat soluble*	*Maintains red blood cells; prevents clotting; essential in cell respiration*	*Vegetable oils, raw seeds and nuts, soybeans*	*10 mg for men and 8 mg for women. Weak muscles; fatigue; bad skin*
Vitamin K	*Fat soluble*	*Proper blood clotting*	*Leafy green vegetables, milk, yogurt, polyunsaturated oils, egg yolks*	*80 mg for men and 65 mg for women. Improper clotting*

MINERALS

Minerals are chemical elements such as calcium, sodium, iron, and magnesium which the body does not manufacture but needs in small amounts for various bodily functions. Like vitamins, minerals are available in many of the foods we eat or in capsule supplements available in health food stores. Table B lists minerals, their function, foods in which they are contained, and consequences of deficiencies.

* International Units

TABLE B

MINERALS	BODILY FUNCTION	FOODS PROVIDING MINERALS	RDA RESULTS OF DEFICIENCY
Calcium	*Builds strong bones and teeth; involved in nerve transmission and muscle contraction; promotes healthy blood, muscle growth, and regulates heartbeat*	*Milk and dairy products, broccoli, tomatoes, oranges, bonemeal*	*800 mg for men and women. Brittle bones, bleeding gums, osteoporosis, nervousness and irritability*
Chromium	*Works with insulin to regulate blood-sugar levels; stimulates enzymes*	*Brewer's yeast, liver, beef, whole-wheat bread, mushrooms*	*50–200 mg for men and women. Poor insulin functioning and glucose intolerance; atherosclerosis*
Copper	*Essential for red blood cell formation, hemoglobin synthesis*	*Liver, whole-grain products, almonds, green leafy vegetables, legumes, seafood*	*1.5–3 mg for men and women. General weakness; poor respiration; bad skin*
Iodine	*Regulates thyroid gland and production of thyroid hormones; promotes growth*	*Seafood (plant and animal), mushrooms, Irish moss, kelp*	*150 mcg for men and women. Lack of vitality; enlarged thyroid; sluggish metabolic rate; goiter*
Iron	*Prevents anemia; necessary for hemoglobin formation; transports oxygen throughout the body; stimulates growth*	*Liver, oysters, heart, leafy green vegetables, whole grains, legumes*	*10 mg for males and 15 mg for females. Anemia (low red blood cell count); low vitality; pallid complexion*

MINERALS	BODILY FUNCTION	FOODS PROVIDING MINERALS	RDA RESULTS OF DEFICIENCY
Magnesium	*Essential for proper heartbeat and nerve transmission; Constituent of bones and teeth*	*Fresh green vegetables, soybeans, milk, corn, apples*	*350 mg for males and 280 mg for females. Weak nervous system and poor muscular control*
Manganese	*Necessary for bone formation, energy production, and protein metabolism*	*Whole-grain cereals, egg yolks, nuts, seeds, green vegetables*	*2.5 mg for males and females. Dizziness; weak bone structure*
Phosphorus	*Assists calcium in maintaining strong bones and teeth; necessary for muscle and nerve function*	*Meat, fish, eggs, poultry, seeds, nuts*	*800 mg for men and women. Poor appetite and weight loss. Bleeding gums*
Potassium	*An electrolyte needed to maintain fluid balance and proper heartbeat; strengthens nervous system*	*All vegetables, oranges, bananas, whole grains, sunflower seeds, mint leaves*	*2000 mg for men and women. Headaches; poor reflexes*
Selenium	*Protects vitamin E; preserves tissue elasticity*	*Brewer's yeast, organ and muscle meats, fish and shellfish, grains, cereals, and dairy products*	*70 mcg for males and 55 mcg for females. Premature aging*
Sodium	*Maintains strong nervous, muscular and lymph systems; Assists potassium in regulating water balance.*	*Seafood, carrots, beets, poultry, meat, and kelp*	*500 mg for males and females*
Sulfur	*Necessary for formation of body tissues*	*Meat, fish, legumes, nuts, eggs, cabbage, dried beans, and brussels sprouts*	*No RDA*

MINERALS	BODILY FUNCTION	FOODS PROVIDING MINERALS	RDA RESULTS OF DEFICIENCY
Zinc	*Component of insulin; required for blood sugar control; aids in digestion; important in wound healing and enzyme activation*	*Meats, poultry, fish, whole-grain products, brewer's yeast, wheat bran, pumpkin seeds*	*15 mg for males and 12 mg for females. Unable to heal quickly*

FATS

Known as lipids, fats are classified as saturated (mostly animal sources) and unsaturated (plant sources). Since carbohydrates are the first source of energy used by the body, fats are stored for long periods of time before they are used as energy. Therefore, high-fat meals cling to the body but do not aid in burning calories. Nevertheless, they cushion the bones and internal organs and provide long-term energy storage, insulation against the cold, and carry the fat-soluble vitamins A, D, E, and K through the blood. Fats are needed in small amounts, and if more calories (measure by fat content) are consumed than needed, there will be weight gain. Fats are contained in meat, cheese, butter, cream, whole-milk products, nuts, olives, avocados, and soybeans.

PROTEIN

Protein, vital for the growth and development of tissues, provides heat and energy, and is the major source for building muscles, blood, skin, hair, nails, and internal organs. A protein deficiency may hinder proper growth, tissue development, and vitality. Additionally, it may be one factor in depression and slow healing of wounds and bruises. During digestion, proteins are broken down into amino acids. In order for the body to properly synthesize protein, amino acids must be present. Of the twenty-two acids, eight are known as essential amino acids and must be obtained from foods. The other fourteen are manufactured by the body. Protein-rich foods which contain amino acids are fish, poultry, meat, eggs, milk, beans, cheese, dried peas, and whole grains. A vegetarian can still get the proper amount of protein using the correct combination of grains and vegetables. While proteins are the main source of building-block materials, an overage is converted to fat and stored for future energy.

CARBOHYDRATES

We get carbohydrates, the body's most immediate source of energy, from sugars, starches, and cellulose (fiber). Especially rich are complex carbohydrates, which include rice, pasta, cereals, potatoes, whole-grain breads, and some fruits and nuts. While complex carbohydrates burn calories quickly, an abundance of refined carbohydrates such as white flour, white sugar, and polished rice should be kept to a minimum since they are lacking B-complex vitamins and fiber.

FIBER

Fiber, or roughage, refers to the undigested portion of grains, fruits, and vegetables, called cellulose, which moves food and its accompanying toxins through the intestines by pulling water into the digestive tract, aiding the elimination process. By decreasing the amount of time stools remain in the bowels, fiber is an important factor for reducing the risk of a plethora of illnesses including colon cancer, heart disease, and diabetes. Whole-grain breads, cereals, fruits, and vegetables are all fiber rich.

Ayurveda

Ayurveda (Sanskrit for "science of life") is an ancient method of healing from India that categorizes us by three distinct personality types, or doshas (Sanskrit for "temperament")—Vata, Pitta, and Kapha—which encompass one's physical and mental condition. Vata is irritable, intolerant, and drawn toward foods, which encourages the buildup of gas. Kapha is slow, depressive, and tends to gain weight, especially since he or she consumes an overabundance of sugar, wheat, and fried foods. Pitta is very quick, nervous, and hot-tempered due to an affinity for caffeine and hot, spicy foods. Ayurvedic doctors agree that most physical conditions are precipitated and agitated by what we eat, exercise or lack of it, our acquired habits and patterns, even the climate in which we live.

Each temperament is drawn to and aggravated by one or more of six categories into which food is divided—pungent, bitter, sour, astringent, sweet, and salty. Foods associated with each of these categories are as follows:

1. *Sweet*—sugar, honey, rice, milk, cream and butter
2. *Salty*—cheese, processed foods, sodium-high food
3. *Sour*—lemons, cheese, yogurt, tomatoes, grapes, plums, vinegar
4. *Bitter*—bitter greens (endive, chicory, romaine lettuce), tonic water, spinach
5. *Pungent*—cayenne, chili peppers, onions, garlic, radishes, ginger, spicy food, curries

6. *Astringent*—beans, lentils, apples, pears, cabbage, broccoli, cauliflower, potatoes[13]

When these foods are eaten to excess, the ailments associated with those doshas are intensified. To allay the symptoms and regain balance and moderation, certain exercises, climactic changes, personality adjustments, and a pacifying diet consisting of foods affiliated with another dosha are recommended. Like other holistic practitioners, the Ayurvedic physician observes the body type, interviews the patient, and reviews the answers to a series of questions relating to habits, likes, dislikes, etc., in order to make a correct diagnosis. Some people may be exclusively one type, but most are a combination of two or three. For instance, you can have a Kapha body, that is, sluggish, heavy, with a slow metabolism, and yet have a Pitta mind, i.e., hot-tempered, aggressive, and mentally alert.

In addition to the zodiacal signs, each planet is associated with a particular dosha as follows:

VATA PLANETS: Mercury, Saturn, and Uranus
PITTA PLANETS: Mars, Sun, and Pluto
KAPHA PLANETS: Venus, the Moon, Jupiter, and Neptune

Knowing the dosha associated with your sun sign, moon sign, and ascendant may help you to assess your Ayurvedic body type(s). If you have a copy of your horoscope, the planets placed on the angles of the chart (See Chapter 1) will also aid in your assessment.

HERBAL REMEDIES

When we think about herbs, what comes to mind are food seasonings (plants, spices, and condiments) that access food's natural flavors, or aromatic, soothing teas. In addition to their culinary uses, fresh or dried herbs are used in compresses or for steaming the face. Oils extracted from plants are great for massage, bathing, and as inhalants.

Wild herbs and spices have been used cosmetically and medicinally for centuries in cultures where they grow. Some herbs grow wild in certain parts of the world and may be difficult to obtain, while others have been transported, cultivated, and can be grown in your garden. Native Americans, for instance, have always utilized goldenseal and echinacea, so-called miracle cures for common colds and flus which the public are only beginning to discover. Even garlic and ginger, which are routinely used to enliven cuisine and have been a part of Chinese food preparation for centuries, are said to contain properties that cleanse the system of impurities. Chamomile, commonly used in tea or facial steam, is considered to be an all-around healing agent which eases inflammations, calms nerves, and helps to release toxins. Herbs such as comfrey, blackberry, and senna can be ingested as tea but must be used wisely since they are powerful and overuse can do more harm than good.

One of the most influential books explaining the healing power of plants and herbs is Nicholas Culpeper's *The Complete Herbal*, originally published in England in 1649 and still utilized as a reference text. A noted herbalist, Culpeper describes the medicinal value of various herbs and plants for treating disease. Since it was commonplace for his contemporaries to utilize astrology to understand their lives, Culpeper also categorized each plant according to sign and planet. In fact, in seventeenth-century Britain, astrology was not merely taught in the universities but accepted by farmers and horticulturalists, who observed that seasonal changes and the positions of the luminaries definitively affected plant growth.

Like Culpeper, some astrologers/herbologists recommend that people born under certain zodiacal signs incorporate specific herbs into their diet. These correlations are arrived at by observing that a particular herb's healing properties may relieve mental and physical conditions that befall those born under a specific zodiacal sign. Other plants have qualities similar to the characteristics of one of the zodiacal signs or planets. An obvious case in point would be chamomile, a known tranquilizer, recommended for Geminis and Aquarians, who tend to be nervous and high-strung.

AROMATHERAPY AND ESSENTIAL OILS

Aromatherapy is the umbrella term for the prevention, treatment, and ultimate healing of certain mental and physical conditions through the use of essential oils, which are obtained from a plant's roots, stalks, flowers, leaves, or fruit. Aromatherapy is experiencing a renaissance; most ancient cultures, including Egyptians, Greeks and Romans, used oil extracts from indigenous herbs and plants extensively, both cosmetically and therapeutically. Essential oils are said to have a profound effect on the nervous system, metabolism, vital organs, and endocrine system and are utilized today to reduce stress and tension by calming the nerves. These extracts can enhance a relaxing bath, add sweet-smelling fragrances to a room, be used as inhalants, or rubbed onto the body.

Haven't you ever walked into a room and immediately responded to a strong odor either positively or negatively? Simplistically speaking, this is how aromatherapy works since strong scents go straight to the hypothalamus, the organ which regulates body temperature, thirst, and hunger. Experiment by placing ten drops of an aromatic oil in hot water or lighting a scented candle at bedtime, making certain to remove any other stimuli, and inhale the scent which pervades the room.

Since a large quantity of plants are required to extract even a minute quantity of oil, certain essential oils are extremely expensive while others are not. Lavender oil is reasonably priced because it is easy to grow and has a high yield of flowers. Conversely, rose oil is very expensive because roses do not produce a large percentage of oil.

Some essential oils are targeted for certain conditions while others can be used as stress relievers for all ailments and personality types. The most commonly used all-purpose essential oils are:

Eucalyptus—Eucalyptus oil is extracted by steam distillation from leaves of the eucalyptus tree, indigenous to Australia and Tasmania. Utilized in commercial rubs and inhalants for chest complaints and colds by easing congestion and opening up breathing passages, its aroma is easily recognizable.

Jasmine—Commonly used in incense, perfume, and potpourri caches, it is a wonderful-tasting tea and an all-purpose relaxant and soother because of its remarkable aroma. If you are extremely nervous, stressed, or anxiety ridden, use jasmine in any form. Expensive when utilized as an oil, it is a perfect remedy for nervous exhaustion and menstrual cramps.

Juniper—Indigenous to Canada and Europe, berries from the juniper bush are used to flavor gin but must be dried and then distilled to create an essential oil. An all-round disinfectant, Juniper can quell cystitis, abdominal pain, menstrual cramps, acne, and anxiety.

Lavender—If in doubt as to which essential oil to choose, lavender, obtained from English and French plants by distillation, is an all-purpose remedy. It is a great antidote for hyperactivity and insomnia and its tranquilizing effects are best utilized as bath oil.

Lemon—Lemon is one of the best all-purpose essential oils as it can be utilized in that form or by squeezing the juice on wounds, bruises, and/or the body part which requires special attention. Massaging lemons on the face, throat, and neck can improve circulation in those areas.

Throughout the book, essential oils which are relevant to a particular physical or emotional condition have been discussed under the zodiacal sign relating to that ailment, as aromatherapy is an extremely useful tool in correcting weaknesses and improving strengths.

ACUPUNCTURE AND ACUPRESSURE

Acupuncture is based on the traditional Chinese theory that the body is made up of meridians—energy pathways that carry a vital life force called *chi* to specific areas and organs. By inserting very thin needles at points along specific meridians where the chi has been blocked, pain is eased and energy restored to the corresponding area of the body. Acupressure massage applies pressure on the meridian points using fingers and thumbs rather than with needles. Whereas acupuncture requires a professional, acupressure can be done by learning which points correspond to the part of the body which is painful, sore, or brittle. Though they may not be a panacea, acupuncture and acupressure may greatly relieve the aches caused by arthritis (a condition resulting from joint inflammation), migraine, and other uncomfortable or distressful ailments. If a backache or headache is determined by the practitioner to be caused by lack of the chi flowing to that part of the body, pain will not only be relieved but may not return.

CHIROPRACTICS

Chiropractic medicine, or spinal manipulation, is based on the premise that many of the body's imbalances, discomforts, and chronic pain are related to posture and its relationship to the nervous system. Chiropractors seek to bring the body into balance through manual manipulation of the spine, joints, and muscles, allowing the neuromusculoskeletal system to function smoothly. Viewed for many years as quackery by the medical establishment, chiropractics is increasingly covered by many insurance plans.

STRESS MANAGEMENT AND RELAXATION TECHNIQUES

The most important way to strengthen the immune system is by learning to cope with stress, that is, remaining cool, calm, and collected in the wake of an emotional storm. For the most part, learning to relax both body and mind before an anxiety attack strikes is the most basic way to head off stress. Channeling your anxiety into exercise, creativity, and general activity is far more productive than indulging in anger, food, alcohol, or drugs, which will only perpetuate, rather than allay, stress. Relaxation techniques include deep breathing, massage, yoga, meditation, visualization, guided imagery, and biofeedback.

Massage Techniques

Massage envelops an assortment of therapies directed at the soft tissues and stimulates the body to utilize its own healing powers. It is a procedure that assists in clearing the mind of stress, treating muscle injuries, reducing swelling, and relieving pain. Massage is regarded as an excellent stress-management tool since so many ailments are either caused or exacerbated by nervous tension. In addition, it can also be utilized to iron out energy blockages, which lead to atrophy, tension, or complete stiffness. It is especially helpful for high-strung, rigid personalities whose illnesses have resulted from this mental state. Different types of massage include:

1. *Swedish massage*—The most common form of stroking, Swedish massage involves gentle muscle manipulation which works on the outer layer of the skin. It is primarily used to ensure relaxation, relieve muscle tension, and improve circulation.

2. *Deep-tissue massage*—Working with stronger pressure to reach deeper layers of muscle, this massage is therapeutic as well as relaxing. If you have constant tension, a stiff neck, or chronic back pain, deep tissue massage may be more suitable. Whereas simple Swedish massage can be done by your partner, deep-tissue massage should be done by a trained masseur or masseuse. If too much pressure is applied or the wrong areas are kneaded, you may do more harm than good.

3. *Acupressure*—Using the same meridians and points as in acupuncture treatment, acupressure is merely acupuncture without needles. Instead of needles, pressure is firmly applied with the fingers so that the chi energy is activated and tension is released.

4. *Shiatsu*—Shiatsu is the Japanese equivalent to acupressure, but utilizing the thumbs. Pressure is applied to the points on the meridians to balance *ki,* the Japanese term for energy. Like acupressure, it relieves blocked energy, promotes good health, and renews vitality.

CREATIVE VISUALIZATION AND GUIDED IMAGERY

These exercises allow an image or series of images to lead you on an imaginary journey to a place where you will be completely relaxed. With your eyes closed and your body in a comfortable position, you will be able to re-create an experience by recalling all its accompanying sensory perceptions. This entails guided imagery techniques under the supervision of a leader who will talk you through a series of events in either a one-on-one or group setting.

If, for instance, lying on a beach is your ideal mode of relaxation, close your eyes, breathe deeply, and imagine that you are surrounded by sun, sand, and the ocean. Remember the last time you visited the beach, and try to once again smell the sand, feel the sunlight on your back, and taste the salt water in your mouth. Remain in that position for a few minutes, slowly open your eyes, and take your time to begin the next activity. Not only will you feel completely relaxed, but you can learn to manage stress if you invoke that feeling every time you become anxious.

BIOFEEDBACK

Biofeedback, a more scientific relaxation technique, involves being hooked up to a machine that monitors pulse and heart rate, blood pressure, and increased perspiration—bodily reactions to stress. By learning to recognize symptoms *before* they result in full-blown ailments such as heart attack, asthma attack, migraine, or other conditions exacerbated by stress, you can control bodily functions such as blood pressure, heart rate, temperature, muscle tension, and brain waves. Biofeedback can be practiced at home with a portable monitor, but the ultimate goal is aimed at recognizing the symptoms before they occur without the help of the machine. Once these signs are identified, relaxation techniques which help to still the mind and body (i.e., deep breathing, visualization, yoga, and meditation) can then be employed to alleviate these symptoms.

YOGA AND MEDITATION

Yoga, Sanskrit for "union of body and mind," encompasses a series of breathing exercises and physical positions called asanas which, when done on a regular basis, stretch, tone, and relax the body, providing comfort to the nervous system and calming the mind. Recorded in the Vedas, Indian books of ancient knowledge, more than two thousand years ago, yogic philosophy propounds that when the body is more supple, energy flows freely, activating different areas of the anatomy. Furthermore, a tranquil mind free of negative impulses will rid the body of stress, thereby empowering the immune system. Throughout this book, various asanas which aid the body part ruled by a particular zodiacal sign have been described.

Combined with meditation (a method of emptying the mind of unwanted, negative thoughts), yoga exercises ultimately help you to become peaceful, relaxed, and tension-free. Meditative techniques which are also done on their own and are used to achieve this goal range from deep breathing, repeating a mantra (set of sounds), chanting, or even a nonthinking activity such as cooking or cleaning. The methods may be different but the serene and stress-free results which are ultimately achieved are the same.

FLOWER ESSENCES

Bach Flower Remedies are homeopathically prepared tinctures of thirty-eight different flower essences categorized according to psychological ailments like fear, anxiety, introversion, etc., which they help to allay. Discovered by Dr. Edward Bach, a British physician, in the 1930s, these thirty-eight varieties are extracted from common herbs like chicory, vervain, water chestnut, agrimony, and vine, which, according to some practitioners, have a subtle but very powerful effect on the psychological state. There are many other groups of essences, e.g., California flower essences and Alaskan flower essences, which are also used medicinally.

Resource Guide

―――― ● ――――

Listing of Health Organizations

Each of the following organizations should be able to refer you to a practitioner in your geographical area.

ALLIANCE FOR ALTERNATIVES IN
  HEALTH CARE
PO Box 6279
Thousand Oaks, CA
  91359–6279
805–494–7818
web site: http://www.alternative
  insurance.com

ALCOHOLICS ANONYMOUS
  WORLD SERVICES
475 Riverside Drive
New York, NY 10163
212–870–3400
web site: http://www.aa.org

AMERICAN CANCER SOCIETY INC.
1599 Clifton Road, N.E.
Atlanta, GA 30329–4251
404–320–3333
web site: http://www.cancer.org

AMERICAN DIABETES
  ASSOCIATION
1660 Duke St.
Alexandria, VA 22314
888–DIABETES
web site: http://www.diabetes.org

AMERICAN HEART ASSOCIATION
7272 Greenville Avenue
Dallas, TX 75231–4596
800–AHA–USA1
800–553–6321 (for information
  about strokes)
web site:
  http://www.americanheart.org

AMERICAN LUNG ASSOCIATION
1740 Broadway
New York, NY 10019
800–LUNG USA
web site: http://www.lungusa.org

ARTHRITIS FOUNDATION
1330 W. Peachtree St.
Atlanta, GA 30309
800–283–7800
web site: http://www.arthritis.org

ASTHMA AND ALLERGY
  FOUNDATION OF AMERICA
1125 15th St., N.W., Suite 502
Washington, DC 20005
800–7ASTHMA
web site: http://www.aafa.org

CROHN'S AND COLITIS
  FOUNDATION OF AMERICA
386 Park Ave. South, 17th Floor
New York, NY 10016–8804
800–932–2423
web site: http://www.ccfa.org

NATIONAL CENTER FOR
  COMPLEMENTARY AND
  ALTERNATIVE MEDICINE
(NCCAM) (affiliated with
  National Institutes of Health)
PO Box 8218
Silver Spring, MD 20907–8218
888–644–6226
Fax 301–495–4957
web site:
  http://www.nccam.nih.gov

NATIONAL HEADACHES
  FOUNDATION
428 W. Saint James Place, 2nd
  Floor
Chicago, IL 60614–2750
800–843–2256
web site:
  http://www.headaches.org

NATIONAL INSTITUTES OF
  HEALTH*
Bethesda, MD 20892
301–496–4000
web site: http://www.nih.gov

NATIONAL KIDNEY FOUNDATION
30 East 33rd Street, Suite 1100
New York, NY 10016
800–622–9010
web site: http://www.kidney.org

NATIONAL OSTEOPOROSIS
  FOUNDATION
150 17th Street, N.W., Suite 500
Washington, DC 20035
202–223–2226
web site: http://www.nof.org

NORTH AMERICAN MENOPAUSE
  SOCIETY
Dept. of OB/GYN
11100 Euclid
Cleveland, OH 44106
216–844–8748
Fax: 216–844–8708
web site:
  http://www.menopause.org

OVEREATERS ANONYMOUS
6075 Zenith Ct., N.E.
Rio Rancho, NM 87124–6424
505–891–2664
web site: http://overeaters
  anonymous.org

WEIGHT WATCHERS
  INTERNATIONAL
175 Crossways Park West
Woodbury, NY 11797
516–390–1400
Fax: 516–677–3755
web site: http://www.weight
  watchers.com

* The National Institutes of Health consists of different institutes specializing in various ailments including cancer, eye diseases, digestive diseases, and diabetes, to name a few. Information on all these can be found on its web site.

Alternative Healing Organizations

Each of the following organizations should be able to refer you to a practitioner in your geographical area.

AMERICAN ACADEMY OF MEDICAL
  ACUPUNCTURE
5820 Wilshire Blvd., Suite 500
Los Angeles, CA 90036
  213–937–5514
web site http://www.medical
  acupuncture.org

AMERICAN ASSOCIATION OF
  ORIENTAL MEDICINE
433 Front St.
Catasauqua, PA 18032
888–500–7999
Fax: 610–264–2768
web site: http://www.aaom.org

AMERICAN ASSOCIATION OF
  NATUROPATHIC PHYSICIANS
601 Valley Street, Suite 105
Seattle, WA 98109
206–298–0126
Fax: 206–298–0129
web site:
  http://www.naturopathic.org

AMERICAN CHIROPRACTIC
  ASSOCIATION
1701 Clarendon Blvd.
Arlington, VA 22209
800–986–4636
web site:
  http://www.amerchiro.org

AMERICAN COLLEGE FOR
ADVANCEMENT IN MEDICINE
23121 Verdugo Drive, Suite 204
Laguna Hills, CA 92653
web site: http://www.acam.org

AMERICAN HERBALISTS GUILD
PO Box 70
Roosevelt, UT 84066
435–722–8434
Fax 435–722–8452
web site: http://www.healthy.net/
  herbalists

AMERICAN HOLISTIC HEALTH
  ASSOCIATION
PO Box 17400
Anaheim, CA 92817–7400
714–779–6152
web site: http://www.ahha.org

AMERICAN ORIENTAL BODYWORK
  THERAPY ASSOCIATION
1000 Whitehorse Rd.
Voorhees, NJ 08043
609–782–1616
web site:
  http://www.healthy.net/aobta

ASSOCIATED BODYWORK AND
  MASSAGE PROFESSIONALS
28677 Buffalo Park Rd.
Evergreen, CO 80439–7347
800–458–2267
web site: http://www.ABMP.com

ASSOCIATION FOR APPLIED
  PSYCHOPHYSIOLOGY AND
  BIOFEEDBACK
10200 W. 44th Ave., Suite 304
Wheat Ridge, CO 80033
800–477–8892
web site: http://www.akpb.org

AYURVEDIC INSTITUTE
11311 Menaul NE
Albuquerque, NM 87112
505–291–9698
Fax: 505–294–7572
web site:
  http://www.ayurveda.com

THE CHOPRA CENTER FOR WELL
  BEING
7630 Fay Avenue
La Jolla, CA 92037
888–424–6772
Fax: 858–551–7811
web site: http://www.chopra.com

The Edward Bach Centre
  (Bach Remedies)
Mount Vernon, Sotwell
Wallingford, Oxon
OX 10 OPZ
England
44–1491–834678

HealthWorld Online
  Professional Referral
  Network
10751 Lakewood Blvd.
Downey, CA 90241
562–862–6116
Fax: 562–862–2893
web site: http://www.healthy.net

International Association for
  Colon Hydrotherapy
PO Box 461285
San Antonio, TX 78246–1285
210–366–2888
Fax: 210–366–2999
web site:
  http://www.healthy.net/iact

National Center for
  Homeopathy
801 N. Fairfax St., Suite 306
Alexandria, VA 22314
703–548–7790
web site: http://www.homeopathy
  home.com

National Guild of Hypnotists
PO Box 308
Merrimack, NH 03054–0308
603–429–9438
web site: http://www.ngh.net

Patience T'ai Chi Association
PO Box 350532
Brooklyn, NY
718–332–3477
web site:
  http://www.patiencetaichi.com

Appendix V

Listing of Astrology Resources

ASTROLOGICAL ORGANIZATIONS

AMERICAN FEDERATION OF ASTROLOGERS (AFA)
PO Box 22040
Tempe, AZ 85285–2040
888–301–7630
web site: www.astrologers.com

ASSOCIATION FOR ASTROLOGICAL NETWORKING (AFAN)
8306 Wilshire Blvd., PMB 537,
Beverly Hills, CA 90211
800–578–AFAN
Fax: 212–932–2446
web site: http://www.afan.org

INTERNATIONAL SOCIETY FOR ASTROLOGICAL RESEARCH (ISAR)
PO Box 38613
Los Angeles, CA 90038–0613
805–525–0461
Fax: 805–933–0301
web site:
http://www.isarastrology.com

NATIONAL COUNCIL FOR GEOCOSMIC RESEARCH (NCGR)
PO Box 38866
Los Angeles, CA 90038
818–761–6433
Fax: 818–505–1440
web site:
http://www.geocosmic.org

ASTROLOGICAL CHART SERVICES

For computerized printout of your horoscope and astrological software programs, contact:

AMERICAN COUNCIL OF VEDIC ASTROLOGY (ACVA)
PO Box 2149
Sedona, AZ 86339
800–900–6595
web site: www.vedicastrology.org

ASTROLABE, INC.
350 Underpass Road
PO Box 1750
Brewster, MA 02631
508–896–5081
Fax: 508–896–5289
web site: http://www.alabe.com

THE ASTROLOGICAL ASSOCIATION OF GREAT BRITAIN (AA)
Unit 168, Lee Valley Technopark
Tottenham Hale, London N17 9LN
U.K.
Phone: 0181–880–4848
web site: www.astrologer.com

ASTROLOGICAL CONSULTING SERVICES

Ronnie Gale Dreyer
PO Box 8034, FDR Station
New York, NY, 10150–8034
212–799–9187
Fax: 212–799–2748
e-mail: RGDreyer@aol.com
web site:
http://members.aol.com/
rgdreyer

BRITISH ASSOCIATION FOR VEDIC ASTROLOGY (BAVA)
19 Jenner Way
Romsey, Hampshire S051 8PD
U.K.
Phone: 01794–524178
web site: www.bava.org

Suggested Reading*

Ajaya, Swami, *Psychotherapy, East and West: A Unifying Paradigm.* Honesdale: Himalayan International Institute of Yoga, Science, and Philosophy of the U.S.A., 1983.

American Heart Association, *The American Heart Association Cookbook.* New York: Ballantine Books, 1991.

Avery, Jeanne, *Astrology and Your Health.* New York: Simon and Schuster, 1991.

Beattie, Melody, *Codependent No More.* New York: Harper/Hazelden, 1987.

Boston Women's Health Book Collective, *The New Our Bodies, Ourselves: A Book by and for Women.* New York: Simon & Schuster, 1984.

Carter and Weber, *Body Reflexology.* New York: Reward Books, 1995.

Chopra, M.D., Deepak, *Perfect Health.* New York: Harmony Books, 1990.

Chopra, M.D., Deepak, *Quantum Healing.* New York: Bantam Books, 1990.

* There are countless books available which are written about astrology as well as the ailments and remedies contained in this book. These are just a portion which I have found extremely helpful.

Culpeper, Nicholas, *Culpeper's Color Herbal* (edited by David Potterton). New York: Sterling Publishing Co., Inc., 1983.

Cunningham, Donna, *An Astrological Guide to Self-Awareness.* York Beach: Samuel Weiser, Inc., 1986.

Cunningham, Donna, *Flower Remedies Handbook.* New York: Sterling Publishing Co., 1992.

Doress-Worters, Paula B. and Diana Laskin Siegal, in cooperation with the Boston Women's Health Book Collective, *The New Ourselves, Growing Older: Women Aging with Knowledge and Power.* New York: Simon & Schuster, 1994.

Dreyer, Ronnie Gale, *Vedic Astrology.* York Beach, ME: Samuel Weiser, Inc., 1997.

Dreyer, Ronnie Gale, *Venus.* Wellingborough, England: Aquarian Press, 1994.

Frawley and David, *Ayurveda and the Mind.* Silverlake, WI: Lotus Light Publications, 1997.

Gawain, Shakti, *Meditations: Creative Visualization and Meditation Exercises to Enrich Your Life.* Novato, CA: New World Library, 1991.

Geddes, Sheila, *Astrology and Health.* Wellingborough, CA: Aquarian Press, 1982.

George, Demetra and Bloch, Douglas, *Astrology for Yourself.* Berkeley, England: Wingbow Press, 1987.

Gorbach, M.D., Sherwood, Zimmerman, David R., and Woods, Margo, *The Doctors' Anti-Breast Cancer Diet.* New York: McGraw-Hill Publishing, 1984.

Grace, Kendra, *Aromatherapy Pocketbook.* St. Paul, MN: Llewellyn Publications, 1999.

Grinberg, Avi, *Foot Analysis: The Foot Path to Self-Discovery.* York Beach, ME: Samuel Weiser, Inc., 1993.

Hittelman, Richard, *Yoga—28 Day Exercise Plan.* New York: Bantam Books, 1973.

Iyengar, B.K.S., *Light on Yoga.* New York: Schocken Books, 1966.

Jarmey, Chris and Tindall, John, *Acupressure for Common Ailments.* New York: Simon & Schuster, 1991.

Jensen, Dr. Bernard, *Foods That Heal*. Garden City, NY: Avery Publishing Group, 1988.

Kloss, Jethro, *Back to Eden*. Loma Linda, CA: Back to Eden Press, 1995.

Knutson, Gunilla, *Book of Massage*. New York: St. Martin's Press, 1972.

Leibowitz, Judith, *The Alexander Technique*. New York: Harper & Row, 1990.

Love, Susan M., *Dr. Susan Love's Breast Book*. Malibu, CA: Perseus Press, 1995.

Love, Susan M., *Dr. Susan Love's Hormone Book: Making Informed Choices About Menopause*. New York: Random House, 1998.

McFarlane, Stewart, *The Complete Book of Tai Chi*. London, New York: Dorling Kindersley, 1997.

Mayo, Jeff, *The Astrologer's Astronomical Handbook*. Essex, England: L. N. Fowler & Co. Ltd., 1982.

Michaels, Jennifer, *What's Your Diet Sign?* New York: McGraw-Hill Publishing Co., 1985.

Mishra, Rammurti, *Fundamentals of Yoga*. London: Lyrebird Press Ltd, 1972.

Nutrition Search, Inc., *Nutrition Almanac*. New York: McGraw-Hill Publishing Co., 1996.

Pascarelli, Emil and Quilter, Deborah, *Repetitive Strain Injury: A Computer User's Guide*. New York: John Wiley & Sons, 1994.

Peck, M. Scott, *The Road Less Traveled*. New York: Simon and Schuster, 1979.

Polunin, Miriam, and Robbins, Christopher, *The Natural Pharmacy*. London: Dorling Kindersley, 1992.

Prevention magazine editors, *The Doctors Book of Home Remedies*. New York: Bantam Books, 1991.

Ridder Patrick, Jane, *A Handbook of Medical Astrology*. London: Penguin Arkana, 1990.

Rogers-Gallagher, Kim, *Astrology for the Light Side of the Brain*. San Diego: ACS Publications, 1996.

Robers-Gallagher, Kim, *Transits for the Light Side of the Future*. San Diego: ACS Publications, 1998.

Sadler, Julie, *Aromatherapy*. London: Ward Lock Villiers House, 1994.

Schwartz, M.D., Jack, *Food Power*. New York: McGraw-Hill Publishing Co., 1979.

Seymour, Percy, *Astrology: The Evidence of Science*. Luton, England: Lennard Publishing, 1988.

Soffer, Shirley, *The Astrology Sourcebook*. Los Angeles: Lowell House, 1998.

Star, Gloria, *Woman to Woman*. St. Paul, MN: Llewellyn Publications, 1999.

Star, Gloria, ed., *Astrology for Women: Roles and Relationships*. St. Paul, MN: Llewellyn Publications, 1997.

Tannen, Deborah, *You Just Don't Understand: Women and Men in Conversation*. New York: William Morrow, 1990.

Tyl, Noel, *Astrological Timing of Critical Illness*. St. Paul, MN: Llewellyn Publications, 1998.

Williams, Jude C., *Jude's Herbal Home Remedies*. St. Paul, MN: Llewellyn Publications, 1992.

Williamson, Marianne, *A Return to Love: Reflections on the Principles of a Course in Miracles*. New York: HarperPerennial, 1996.

End Notes

1. *The Evidence of Science,* Dr. Percy Seymour, p. 12.
2. *Perfect Health,* Deepak Chopra, p. 300.
3. *Perfect Health,* Deepak Chopra, p. 41.
4. *Repetitive Strain Injury: A Computer User's Guide,* Emil Pascarelli and Deborah Quilter, p. 31.
5. *Repetitive Strain Injury: A Computer User's Guide,* Emil Pascarelli and Deborah Quilter, pp. 26, 160, and 177.
6. *Consumer Guide to Alternative Medicine: In Consultation with the American Association of Naturopathic Physicians,* p. 406.
7. *Acupressure for Common Ailments,* Chris Jarmey and John Tindall, p. 25.
8. *Aromatherapy,* Julie Sadler, pp. 56–57.
9. *The Doctors Book of Home Remedies,* Prevention Editors, Bantam, p. 377.
10. *The Doctors Book of Home Remedies,* Prevention Editors, Bantam, p. 217.
11. *Aromatherapy,* Julie Sadler, p. 41.
12. *Body Reflexology,* Carter and Weber, Reward Books, p. 1.
13. *Perfect Health,* Deepak Chopra, pp. 236–41.

Index

ABOUT THE AUTHOR

RONNIE GALE DREYER is an internationally known astrological consultant, lecturer, and teacher based in New York City. She is the author of *Vedic Astrology: A Guide to the Fundamentals of Jyotish, Your Sun and Moon Guide to Love and Life, Venus: The Evolution of the Goddess and Her Planet,* and a contributor to *Astrology for Women,* Llewellyn's Moon Sign Books, and *Hindu Astrology Lessons.* Ronnie's popular columns and articles have appeared in *Nyon* magazine, *American Astrology* magazine, and *Mountain Astrologer,* and she served as editorial consultant on New Age and self-help books for several major publishing companies. She is presently the editor of the bimonthly member letter for NCGR (National Council for Geocosmic Research).

Ronnie holds a bachelor of arts degree in English/Theater Arts from the University of New Mexico, and studied Vedic astrology, known in Sanskrit as Jyotish, both privately and at Sanskrit University in Benares, India. She cofounded the first astrological computer service in the Netherlands, where she lived for ten years and was the official Dutch representative for Astro*Carto*Graphy. She was secretary of the Association for Astrological Networking (AFAN) from 1992 to 1998, and is presently its presiding officer. Ronnie is on the board of directors of ACT (Astrological Conference on Techniques) and the staff of the New York Astrology Center. She has won several awards for her contributions to the astrological community.

Ronnie has an international clientele, lectures extensively for astrology groups, and conducts ongoing courses and workshops throughout the country. Ronnie has been on the faculty of major national and international conferences, including UAC (United Astrology Congress), the largest gathering of its kind, and has lectured in Canada, Germany, the Netherlands, England, Scotland, Ireland, and Australia. Ronnie is well versed in alternative healing and women's health issues, which she incorporates into her consulting practice.